A *Different*

KIND OF

HEALTH

FINDING *Well-Being* DESPITE ILLNESS

BLAIR JUSTICE, PH.D.

FOREWORD BY

NAOMI JUDD

HOUSTON

1998

2402 Westgate, Suite 200
Houston, Texas 77019–6608
telephone: 713–528–6680
fax: 713–528–6577
peakbook@flash.net

Cover and text design: Nita Ybarra

9 8 7 6 5 4 3 2 1

FIRST EDITION
Printed in the United States of America
Printed on recycled paper.

Library of Congress Cataloging-in-Publication Data

Justice, Blair.
A different kind of health : finding well-being despite illness /
Blair, Justice : foreword by Naomi Judd. — 1st ed.
p.   cm.
Includes bibliographical references and index.
ISBN 09605376-4-3
1. Holistic medicine.   2. Health.   3. Mind and body.
4. Spiritual healing.   I. Title.
R733.J87   1998
610—DC21   97–42433
CIP

To the Memory of Liz,
to Cindy and David,
and, again, to Rita

BOOKS BY BLAIR JUSTICE, PH.D.

A Different Kind of Health: Finding Well-Being Despite Illness
Who Gets Sick: How Beliefs, Moods, and Thoughts Affect Your Health
The Abusing Family (with Rita Justice, Ph.D.)
The Broken Taboo (with Rita Justice, Ph.D.)
Violence in the City

Contents

---✳---

✳

---

*T*here's no such thing as a coincidence. It's just God's way of staying invisible. It's no coincidence you've picked up this book. The message inside can change your life. It sure changed mine.

I'm a member of "the remission society," a rapidly expanding community made up of people who are living with chronic diseases and various medical conditions but still have a sense of well-being and health in spite of our infirmities. Dr. Blair Justice's *A Different Kind of Health* shows how this is possible.

This book provides the evidence on how a growing number of people like me can consider themselves healthy, although their medical records show they have a disease. It tells how it is possible for a sense of well-being and illness to coexist and for joy to be experienced despite pain. I strongly believe *A Different Kind of Health* has a wonderful, well-documented message for all who are infirm, disabled, or otherwise chronically ill. It is not only well-documented and clearly written but is also moving and inspiring.

This is the second book I feel Blair has written just for me. The first, *Who Gets Sick: How Beliefs, Moods, and Thoughts Affect Your Health*, helped save my life. *A Different Kind of Health* helps me to see how I will stay well no matter what happens to me physically.

Let me tell you the story of how Blair came into my life. Some of you may know that in 1990 I was diagnosed with a life threatening liver disease and told that I might have just a few years to live. I was terrified, confused, and ill. The shocking diagnosis and prognosis seemed hideously unfair. After a hard life, I'd finally figured some things out and was actually seeing my dreams come true. Now a doctor in a white lab coat was somberly interpreting tests that spelled an abrupt and miserable end.

As a Registered Nurse, I felt betrayed that medical science offered no answers for the Hepatitis C I had gotten from a needle stick working in ICU. But other answers arrived the day after the physician gave me the grim prognosis. A friend sent me a copy of *Who Gets Sick* by Blair Justice, Ph.D. As I read it, curled up in a fetal position on my bed, it began giving me something medicine hadn't offered . . . hope.

In *Who Gets Sick,* Blair explained with carefully documented scientific research how healing comes from inside while cure comes from the outside. Blair's credentials were impeccable. He is an award-winning former science writer and now a psychobiologist and professor at the University of Texas School of Public Health. As I read the book, I consciously considered for the first time the spirit/mind/body connection. I've always known that we are first and foremost spiritual beings in a physical body and that God is a supernatural being. Now I had evidence presented with research, statistics, and case histories to support my faith in healing. The book made clear that what I knew on an intuitive level was indeed fact—that the mind influences the body. I understood how germs aren't the only cause of disease, that health is much more than an absence of disease, and how the quality of our relationships may have more to do with how often we get sick and how soon we get well than do genes, diet, and other factors. Now I knew I could do something to help myself heal and influence the outcome of my disease. This sent me on a remarkable voyage of self-discovery and a fulfilling journey to wholeness.

I wanted to meet the man who had helped launch me on this journey. On the Farewell Tour with my singing partner/daughter Wynonna, I called Blair's office to invite him to our concert at the Astrodome in Houston, where he lived, so that I could personally thank him. I told him my name. "You say you're the Judge?" he asked over the phone. "No, sir. We're a singing duo called The Judds." It seemed unusual to find someone in Texas who didn't listen to country music but a refreshing surprise not to be known. Blair declined my offer to attend the show until he found out I had Hepatitis C. Ever the scientist, he was curious to see how I was going to entertain for an hour, standing, dancing, and singing.

That night at the Astrodome we set a new attendance record. Our security guards escorted Blair and his lovely psychologist wife Rita into the van with us and then out onto our bus. I was impressed that Blair wasn't impressed by all this hoopla. Instead, he showed his caring spirit in asking how I was handling my illness and the impending loss of my beloved career. He teased, "I know what you're doing up there on stage in this Farewell Tour. You're using the love and support from these fans to stimulate your beleaguered immune system." Bingo! He'd nailed me.

And so our friendship began. Blair has since kept up with me and even contributed to the Naomi Judd Research and Education Fund of the American Liver Foundation. Because I feel responsible any time I endorse someone's work, it's important for me to get to know the person. I've hung out with and supported some pioneering healers and health researchers: Andrew Weil, Deepak Chopra, Joan Borysenko, Rachel Remen, and Candace Pert. Blair Justice is the quiet, unassuming academician among them. You probably won't see him on talk shows, so it's important you read this book.

On the bus at the Astrodome back on February 22, 1991, I predicted to Blair and Rita that I would get well. Now I am indeed a member of the remission society. During that same visit, I also offered to write the Foreword to Blair's next book, and now I happily have that opportunity.

A Different Kind of Health needs to be read by everyone. Anyone who is ill or deals with the sick can find vital information and a path to well-being in it. We have come a long way in proving and understanding the spirit/mind/body connection, and Blair's work has helped the process. The solid foundation on which our growing knowledge is based must continue to be provided by men and women with credentials and personal integrity, like Blair.

Blair Justice has hit a grand slam home run for us all to cheer with this book. His candid revelations of his own tragedies and struggles, alongside moving stories of others who have found "a different kind of health," make this a highly readable and moving book. Buy it. Read it. Pass it around. It may not save your life, but it can certainly help you transform the quality of how you live right to the end.

PREFACE

✸

... To all who are about to read this book ...
may we find and become aware
of the truth in ourselves.

—ECKHART

I wrote *A Different Kind of Health* because I was surprised to discover that many persons with chronic disease or disability gain a sense of well-being in the very presence of their disorder. I was struck by their conviction that life is good despite persistent pain. They have found health at a deeper level than the physical and are able to feel well inside themselves although they know they have a disease or disability. How they come to gain this different kind of health, this well-being, is a theme of the book. In effect, they make themselves bigger than their problem—their pain or disorder—rather than the problem being bigger than they are.

Because there are now thousands, if not millions, of the "sick but well" among the elderly, among those with chronic and recurring illnesses, such as cancer and AIDS, and among disabled persons, a re-examination of what constitutes health is taking place.

Researchers have surprisingly discovered in recent years that inner health, our own sense of well-being, is a more accurate predictor of our mortality than are examinations by physicians and laboratory tests. This finding adds to the evidence showing that our subjective reality, more than objective conditions of our life, strongly influences both the quantity and quality of our years. For more than three decades, research has been establishing that objective indicators—such as where we live, how much money we make, how educated we are, how big our house is, how many cars we have—are poor predictors of whether we live a life of satisfaction. The people in this book have found satisfaction and a way of feeling well inside themselves, although their objective condition is one of illness or disability.

What I know about this different kind of health comes from several sources. One is my experience directing a pilot project to study the effects of imagery and support on the immune system in women who recently completed treatment for breast cancer. Many reported health in the presence of disease. This is a finding I have since come across repeatedly in the growing scientific literature on self-perceived health. As a psychologist, I have also had the opportunity to work in therapy with people who discovered a sense of well-being while in pain. In the community service work I do at hospice I have seen people healed while dying.

Last, what I know about this subject is also from my own life. I am one of the wounded but well people who are in this book. I have lived with pain, both physical and emotional, and disease. My own story is woven into the larger one I present on the ways people come to discover, while ill, a health inside themselves and how it enables them to live with a sense of joy and peace.

A Different Kind of Health is for all those who have ever wondered whether they can be well again, to be able to enjoy life while living or dying with disease or disability. The people in this book are real, their stories are true. Where I have used first names only, they are pseudonyms to preserve patient confidentiality.

—BLAIR JUSTICE

Chapter One

BEING WELL

INSIDE

OURSELVES

For nothing can be sole or whole
That has not been rent.

—W. B. YEATS

That's right. I am quite well.

—PLINY THE YOUNGER

A different kind of health applies to all the people who say, "I'm well although I have something wrong with me." They mean "I'm well *in my life,* and in my being, but I know my body is sick." Because of illness or disability they reach deep inside themselves to find ways to be whole.

There are people undergoing treatment for cancer who describe themselves as healthy and those with other painful, chronic illness who define their health as "good." There are persons confined to wheelchairs because of serious injury or some debilitating disorder who consider themselves "well." Researchers are re-examining what health is in the light of emerging new evidence based on those who feel whole despite disease. I am among many with this different kind of health.

The evidence is showing that those of us who have a record of physical pathology but also a *subjective* sense of health acknowledge our condition and the implications of our disorder but feel well at a deeper level of the self than the physical. We simply define our health differently.[1] This different definition is finding support in more than just psychological studies. It is based on the proper measure of health as being not the absence of disease but a sense of well-being, a definition the U.S. Surgeon General has endorsed.[2] Well-being means having "a deep and abiding sense that, despite the day's woes," life is good. "Even when the surface waters churn, the deep currents run sure."[3]

The impetus for scientists to re-examine what health is first emerged from evidence dating back to the early 1980s showing that what we believe about our own health is a powerful predictor of how long we will live—the number of years we have remaining—and how well we will live—the quality of our lives.[4] In fact, it predicts our longevity more accurately than do clinical assessments based on physical examinations by physicians and laboratory tests.[5] There is evidence, then, that subjective health—our own self-perception of being a sick or well *person*—is more important than objective health, a finding that directly violates biomedicine's long-standing definition of what health is.

What is even more intriguing is that many who perceive themselves as being healthy also experience pain and medical problems on a daily basis. What is becoming apparent to clinical investigators is that when people rate their own health, they are telling us not only how they feel about their lives but also about how they experience themselves at a core level of self.[6] They are talking about the quality of their whole life and their experience of a nonphysical well-being.[7] It is our nonphysical self that can enliven us in the face of physical failure and give us the spirit that makes us feel vital and well in our essence.

Many of those who have infirmities or impairments, myself included, regard health as being attainable in places beyond the body.[8] I spent many years believing that health—the degree to which I felt whole, hale, hardy (all meanings of the word)—depended on the extent I was free of pain. I have learned that well-being, being well inside myself, may be related to my physical status but is not dependent on it—any more than happiness is dependent on material wealth. As we will see in Chapter 2, well-being comes from experiences that take us beyond ourselves and connect us with a larger identity and wholeness.

There is "a new way of being whole" and well, as Topf and Bennett put it.[9] Linda Noble Topf's experience with progressive multiple sclerosis has led her to discover that with "a slight shift in perception," one can have a sense of being intact and undiminished "that makes life better, whether the disease gets better or not."[10]

A woman undergoing treatment for metastatic cancer said: "I am really very healthy. I just have this problem, but I am still me."[11] When we perceive the essence of our "me-ness"—who we are— on a level deeper than the body, our self-integrity as a whole remains intact, and we can still feel alive and well.

OUR BELIEFS AND LONGEVITY

Mind moves matter.

—VIRGIL

But how can our own sense of health have an effect on the length of our lives? Even if people are able to draw on "very important internal information" that escapes the best of diagnostic and prognostic assessment,[12] how is it possible that a subjective state of health can influence a very real, objective event such as mortality? The answer is that belief affects biology, sometimes very strongly. The power of belief to influence our physical health is well-established in scientific literature.[13]

For example, when patients believe in the doctors attending them, they get well faster.[14] If an anesthetist visits a patient the night before surgery and succeeds in establishing rapport and trust, less anesthesia will be required the next day and recovery is speeded up.[15] People optimistic about their health have been shown to have a significantly lower risk of premature death.[16]

In psychotherapy, when we change our self-defeating beliefs about ourselves and the way the world is we improve, and changes occur in the limbic system of our brain that are similar to those produced by therapeutic drugs.[17] When we believe that life is good and, despite pain and trauma, "all is or will be well," we live longer and enjoy life more.[18] Even in the final stages of terminal illness, when people strongly believe they will live to participate in some special occasion—an anniversary, birthday, religious observance—the statistics show they do.[19]

The heart is a prime example of how our body is affected by our mind. It is both a mechanical pump and an organ deeply influenced by emotion. Hostility, cynicism, pessimism, depression, and anxiety are all well-documented feelings and attitudes that undermine the health of the heart and cardiovascular system.[20] There is truth, then, in the poetic notion that the heart is the seat of love and compassion as well as in the scientific view that it is a pumping mechanism.[21]

The evidence that the beliefs we have about our own health predict how much longer we have to live comes from an impressive number of good studies. Two researchers, one at Rutgers University, the other at Yale University School of Medicine, reviewed longitudinal studies on thousands of people in this country, Canada, and abroad. Drs. Ellen Idler and Stanislav Kasl concluded that "self-evaluations of health"—whether we perceive ourselves as sick or well—"predict mortality, above and beyond . . . the presence of health problems, physical disability, and biological or life-style risk factors."[22] In other words, regardless of whether we have a disease or not, the belief we have about ourselves and our health—our sense of health—is a key factor in the length of our lives.

ON THE OTHER SIDE OF PAIN

For all happiness mankind can gain
Is not in pleasure, but in rest from pain.
—DRYDEN

A subjective sense of health involves an inner knowing that Western medicine is skeptical of, although such knowledge has long been accepted by cultures steeped in Eastern traditions and practices. Just as we may have an inner sense of health, we also may have intuitive knowledge of imminent death although our medical condition gives no hint of any serious condition. Not infrequently Buddhist priests, for example, will announce their own impending deaths, even when all objective indicators show no sign of ill health or imminent demise.[23] In Western scientific literature well-documented evidence tells of healthy New Guinea clansmen who die because they believe they have violated a sacred taboo.[24] They withdraw, give up their sense of health, and quickly die. At the other end of the spectrum are people who are sick, even dying, who discover they have an inner health and strength and use it to prolong life.

Sickness and pain are a universal aspect of human experience, but we know next to nothing about how people come to experience a sense of health in the presence of illness. On any given day, only 12 percent of the general population report having no pain or other symptoms.[25] When surveys are made of the U.S. population, 50 percent of us have "a medical condition on any given day."[26] Yet 80 percent of us rate ourselves as "well" or healthy.[27] Clearly we have a different kind of health than the one physicians look for in their examinations of us.

What is remarkable about these findings is that so little has been written on the ways that we are well, on what it is inside us that we experience as healthy even when the external evidence shows we have physical problems. Although the prevalence of chronic disease and disorder is increasing as we live longer in this country, medical researchers have scarcely reported on what leads many people to perceiving themselves as having a subtle inner strength, which never shows up on medical charts. The people I present in this book will help answer the question of how the sick can be well. The answer, as we will see, is that they find ways to become part of something bigger than the self, something whole and healthy they internalize that gives them an enthusiasm for life, a sense of involvement and belonging.

OUR UNRECOGNIZED STRENGTH

A remedy too strong for the disease.

—SOPHOCLES

An inner light will shine forth from us.

—GOETHE

Many persons with chronic illness or pain are never asked how they manage to carry on their lives quite effectively though sick or impaired. Dr. Robert Shuman, a practicing psychologist who was diagnosed with multiple sclerosis in 1982, believes that "all too often, patients are told what a sickness *should* mean for them—in terms of treatment, disability, changes in lifestyle. Objectively, such an assessment may be accurate. If, however, it does not speak to the felt truth of the patient's experience, it is useless" or worse.[28] Quadriplegics are seldom asked—even by doctors who treat them—what it is like to live and function without functional use of limbs.[29] Persons who are disabled or chronically ill often have a resilience and strength that goes unrecognized in the medical statistics on disease and disorder. Clinical science has focused so narrowly on what is wrong with us that it has sorely neglected what is also right about us.

What's right about us is the power of what has been termed in the medical literature our *subjective state of health*[30] or what I call our inner health. We discover we have it when we develop our nonphysical sense of self and make it prominent in our lives. We discover it when we come to realize that aspects of our self extend far beyond, and deeper, than the body, the site of our illness and pain, and connect us to powerful resources of health that give us a basic identity of being whole. In discovering our inner health we change how we look at our condition, our pain, so that we think about it in a way that affirms life rather than negates it. We respond to illness differently, depending on who we are, what we believe, and what we learn from infirmity. As Shuman points out:

> Illness is an event that makes a painful difference in the world we take for granted. For some people, their lives are irrevocably damaged. For others, the cracks in their world are patched up. And there are those for whom a former world falls apart and something new replaces the old.[31]

REMISSION SOCIETY AND PAIN FELLOWSHIP

Those who do not feel pain

seldom think that it is felt.

—SAMUEL JOHNSON

Fortunately, more research is now being done on the rapidly expanding community of people who are living with chronic diseases and various medical conditions—from cancer and heart disease to arthritis and disabilities of aging to diabetes and depression. Within that league of the sick or wounded, there are a large number who are functionally well. As long as we carry out our activities of daily living, many of our wounds are invisible to others. Dr. Arthur Frank, the sociologist who wrote of his experience with cancer and a heart attack, calls this growing community of copers "the remission society."[32] Those in the remission society join with the many who cannot carry on daily activities to make up what Albert Schweitzer called the "Fellowship of Those Who Bear the Mark of Pain."[33] One out of three people has some form of chronic pain.

The legions who belong to this community and fellowship have medical records that show the objective presence of active or inactive disease or disorder, which constitutes some kind of pathology or alteration in the cells and tissues of our bodies or brains. I have a record of cancer, depression, injury, and abdominal pain, each of which are examples of the recurring or chronic conditions found in the ever-growing society of those with disabilities or debilitating illness.

HEALTH AND DISEASE COEXISTING

Thou shalt not be tempested, thou
shalt not be travailed; thou
shalt not be dis-eased . . .
Thou shalt not be overcome.

—JULIANA OF NORWICH

Traditionally, health and illness have been considered as being on opposite ends of a continuum.[34] This concept has some validity for individuals with acute illnesses, who can be "placed at varying points along this health-illness continuum, and are expected to work their way back towards health."[35] But it "clearly excludes individuals with chronic conditions for whom 'cure' or a return to prediagnosis conditions is not possible, yet who are still able to perform their social roles."[36] It also excludes all those who have a life-threatening or debilitating illness and cannot perform daily roles but who have a sense of well-being and wholeness despite their disease or disability. These are the persons who have said to me, as to other health professionals, "I feel healthy inside but outside I know I am sick."

Those who do not fit the longstanding medical concept that a person is either sick or well, but never both, have been left dangling in a noncategory of "liminality."[37] In a certain sense, the wounded but well are at the border between two realms of the self, the nonphysical and physical, and have chosen the first for their health. In Celtic times, such a frontier or border was referred to as a "limen," designating "places that stand between spiritual and temporal realms," between the sacred and secular.[38] It is at these "thin places," where we cross from the physical to the nonphysical parts of the self, that we have the opportunity to find a different kind of health.

No Contradiction

Life is both dreadful and wonderful . . .

—THICH NHAT HANH

For those, then, in the remission society and pain fellowship who have found a wholeness beyond the temporal, it isn't a contradiction to say health and disease can coexist.[39] It is a contradiction only if health is considered to mean that no objective sign of pathology can be detected,[40] which is not what health means to people who experience having it. For them health and disease are not binary opposites.

Delores, one of the women in the breast cancer study we conducted at the University of Texas–Houston School of Public Health in collaboration with M.D. Anderson Cancer Center is an example of the many who contradict the medical definition of health.[41] She says she has good health, despite the fact that she has metastases to the spine and shoulders.[42]

"I know that health is supposed to be something that means you are disease-free," she said, " but that definition doesn't fit me." Delores said she feels good and is capable of doing things that "aren't real hard; I just can't push and pull like I used to." She takes care of herself as well as three children, all teenagers. "To me, health includes mental and spiritual health, which I think I have." Thus, she has a strong sense of inner well-being, which is the core of health. As one physician has commented:

A sense of being "healthy"... is dependent not on the presence or absence of disease, but on a sense of being able to 'live fully,' often in spite of physical infirmity. Indeed, some claim that they feel "healthier" since their diagnosis, due to changes in priorities, relationships, insight, or mortality confronted.[43]

But the shift in thinking of health as a negative—the absence of something—to a positive—being fully alive or well inside—has been slow to occur. Many public health scientists, looking at the health of populations, still define health in terms of death rates while a number of clinical researchers continue to regard it as a negative state. This is true despite the World Health Organization's insisting since 1970 that health is more than the absence of disease, that it is a state of physical, emotional, and social well-being.[44] In 1991, the U.S. Surgeon General and the Public Health Service itself declared that health is "best measured" by a "sense of well-being."[45]

HEALTH AS WELL-BEING

He made her melancholy, sad, and heavy;

and so she died; had she being light like you,

of such a merry, nimble, stirring spirit,

she might ha' been a grandma ere she died;

and so may you, for a light heart lives long.

—SHAKESPEARE

The hard evidence in support of this shift to a new definition began accumulating when survey researchers started asking people

to rate their own health. Up to 80 percent of the population, including many with diagnosed medical conditions, see themselves as
in excellent or good health.[46] A much smaller percent with no
physical pathology see themselves as in poor health.[47] It became
apparent that a number of "well" people (by medical standards) are
not healthy and many others with diagnosed disorders believe
themselves healthy.

In the group of the well but sick are those who recover from a
myocardial infarction and have a complete healing of the heart
muscle and normal cardiac functioning but insist they are ill and
cannot carry on activities of daily living.[48] In the sick but well
community are those with chronic conditions who have pathology
but are vital, inspirited human beings.

On Dr. Larry Dossey's first day as an intern on a medical ward
he encountered a patient in a wheelchair who looked very sick,
but he was told by a resident physician that nothing was wrong
with the man. "That's old Hunter," the resident said, "nothing at all
the matter with him."[49] When he was in his thirties, Hunter had
begun to experience chest pain. Every conceivable test proved normal. But Hunter's belief that he had heart disease grew, and as his
conviction increased so did his disability. He became crippled by it.
Before he became disabled, he had worked as a butcher but he quit
because he was convinced that physical exertion would make his
pain worse and lead to a heart attack. "He gradually receded into
inactivity, focusing on the pain which no one could demonstrate as
'real,'" but it was so real it finally confined his life to a wheelchair.

The resident instructing Dossey commented: "His hospital
record's volumes thick. All normal numbers. A real monument to
ol' Hunter's health."[50] Health? To Dossey, still trying to learn the
ropes of being a doctor, the thought was absurd. Even to an intern,
"the objective and subjective meanings of health seemed dis-
crepant."[51] Later, Dossey decided that "health will never be ade-
quately described by numbers alone, or by fat charts detailing

normal studies. Hunter was right and we were wrong. He *was not* healthy, and he knew it." In this case, physicians were insisting health is present when it was not.

In the case of John, the oldest patient Dossey had once he entered private practice, health was not present by medical standards when in fact it was present. "All the nurses and physicians in my medical group knew and loved him dearly," Dossey said.[52] Every time he visited my office for an appointment the entire clinic buzzed with excitement, for it was a remarkable experience to see him and talk to him....He never complained. He smiled much, even laughed, and seemed immune to his many ailments."

John had to have an artificial pacemaker implanted because of heart failure, and the surgical incision became infected. Then the infection spread to the blood. He developed pneumonia, and his kidneys failed. "And there he lay, still alive on morning rounds in the critical care unit, most of his major organ systems artificially supported and poorly functioning except one: his brain. As usual, and for reasons I could not explain, he was intensely alert, even chipper." Dossey tried to find something encouraging to tell John and saw that his failed kidneys had produced a meager amount of urine. He said, "John, your kidneys started working again; you're better." John smiled and replied: "Thank you doctor. Now tell me: Better than what?" Dossey said:

> As I stood there I was taken with a thought that made no sense at the time: *This man is healthy.* Lying helplessly, affixed to various gadgets, this gentle, wise, alert man seemed *beyond* the distinctions of health and illness. John seemed to transcend the easy classifications of "sick or well," "better or worse." And he *knew* it, too—he *experienced* this transcendence, radiating a kind of healthiness even while moribund. An hour later John died—I am convinced, in good health.[53]

THE POWER OF PERCEIVED HEALTH

The mind is its own place, and in itself,
Can make a heaven of hell, a hell of heaven.

—MILTON

Clinical observations, then, as well as empirical studies, have steadily mounted confirming that people can have disabilities from age, illness, or injury and possess a perceived health that predicts survival better than standard clinical assessments. This is not to dismiss the value of medical tests. There *is* a correlation between self-perceived health and what tests show, but the stronger predictor of mortality is our subjective sense.[54] Those who are sick by medical standards but well inside themselves simply have a different kind of health. It is powerful in its effects and should give new hope to the 100 million Americans who have chronic conditions.

The vast majority of us will not die, as our grandparents did, of an acute illness such as pneumonia or tuberculosis or some other infectious disease for which there is now a cure. Most of us today will approach the end of our lives with chronic conditions we have had for a number of years. Drs. Lois Verbrugge and Donald Balaban, gerontology researchers, note that "one's sense of well-being and physical symptoms from a chronic condition . . . are dynamic. They fluctuate over time in response to disease activity and to medical and personal interventions."[55]

Our symptoms also fluctuate in response to how we feel about ourselves, our conditions, and the quality of our life. Studies now indicate that our cognitions, our beliefs about our lives and our health, exert strong influence on whether we actually become disabled or impaired.

OUR PERCEPTIONS AND PAIN

If the doors of perception were cleansed,

everything would appear . . . as it is, infinite.

—BLAKE

What determines our becoming disabled is not simply the severity of our illness or injury; it is also how we perceive ourselves and our condition.[56] Because our beliefs affect not only our psychological well-being but our physical processes as well, we have some control over what disease does to us. A woman I have known and worked with in therapy groups made such a discovery.

Kim Nelson is an attractive, vivacious young woman who has had rheumatoid arthritis since she was 5 years old. She never believed she could climb a mountain. She never believed she could be a "physical" person. "I hated gym class and dreaded anything that required something from my body," she said.[57] As a child, her right knee became chronically inflamed and stiff, a development that led to a diagnosis of rheumatoid arthritis. When she was 12, a cataract was detected in her right eye. In her mid-twenties she was chronically tired and in a bad marriage, which she eventually left.

Kim was still having trouble with her swollen knee and arthritis when she came to a therapy workshop that I conducted with my wife, Rita, a clinical psychologist, in the Colorado Rockies. During her four days with us, she discovered not only what a powerful effect belief has on the body but also how to tap into a sense of inner health she never knew she had.

Kim came to the Rockies believing she had to get rid of her disease to enjoy life. She was surprised by the advice I offered, which was "let your pain sing," a line I borrowed from playwright

Arthur Miller, who said: "Everyone has agony. The only difference is I take my agony and try to make it sing."[58] She believed her pain and her inflamed knee made it impossible to climb the mountain that the group was assigned on the last full day of the workshop. As she slowly trudged up the mountain, trailing the others, Kim began to change her belief.

> Rita helped me take one step at a time by showing me how to enjoy every step. I learned about the wildflowers—how to experience them by smelling and touching them and just being with them. The more I was able to feel with my body, the more my pain would "sing!" By the time we reached the top of the mountain I was crying. I felt my body release both emotional and physical pain. I had never felt so alive.[59]

Going back down the mountain, Kim was in the lead group, letting herself slide like a kid across snowfields. She couldn't believe her pain and knee were letting her enjoy life with such freedom. Kim's identity shifted from pain and illness to an inner sense of health and strength. She discovered her health when she connected to a wholeness beyond the body, to the flowers and mountain, to the group that sang with her, and to a new and deeper sense of being well inside herself.

The perceptions Kim changed about herself, her disease, and her pain have had lasting effects on her body. She discontinued all medication within four months after the workshop, and her knee lets her climb mountains now whenever she wants. She is devoted to being "physical" in her life, moving her body instead of keeping it as immobile as possible. "Ironically, it was after I adopted this new way of thinking that my illness started to lift and leave," she said.[60] (See more on making pain sing in Chapter 6).

CONTROL OVER BEING IMPAIRED

If we have chronic pain and tap into our inner health, as Kim Nelson did, we are likely to find that both our pain and its cause diminish. If we have chronic pain and think of ourselves as disabled because of it, we will experience greater pain and disability.[61]

The more strongly we believe something, good or bad, the more effect there will be on our physiological processes.[62] Thus, optimistic convictions about our health and survival are likely to have a positive effect and pessimistic beliefs a negative one. Emotions are closely linked to strong beliefs and affect our biological functions through the autonomic nervous system and neuro-endocrine pathways.

Dr. John Riley and his colleagues at Brown University have found that patients who believe pain implies impairment are more likely to become impaired.[63] Because pain is ubiquitous and subject to change and relief, except perhaps in some intractable terminal cases, we are better off remaining "optimistic cheerleaders for life at heart"[64] than believing pain means impairment.

Dr. Harold Koenig, a clinical researcher at Duke University Medical Center has studied how "objective chronic illness" gets translated into disability by "how patients perceive themselves and by their world view."[65] Stanford University researchers have also concluded that "with appropriate social and individual behavioral measures, people...can live lives of vitality till very close to the end of their biologically allotted span of years."[66]

These findings should provide encouragement to all of us with chronic or recurring illness. Of the 33 million Americans who are "functionally limited" by a serious condition—arthritis, hypertension, cancer, depression, cardiovascular disease, digestive problems, pain—9 million cannot work, attend school, or maintain a household.[67] The U.S. Public Health Service estimates that 70 percent of the almost 1 trillion dollars spent annually on health care goes to the treatment of these individuals. And "as the population grows older, such conditions will continue to consume an even larger proportion of national health care expenditures."[68]

The evidence now suggests that enormous savings not only in dollars but in improved quality of life can be realized by methods proven to be effective in keeping the severely and chronically ill from becoming disabled. Religious faith, Koenig's research at Duke shows, is one of these modalities.[69] In a large study of persons age 65 or more, Idler and Kasl found that religious involvement not only has a protective effect against disability but, among those who already are impaired, is associated with a higher level of functioning.[70] The more we discover our nonphysical self, the more we can have some effect on the physical.

WE'RE ALL IN THE REMISSION SOCIETY

This life . . . is but an inn,
And we the passengers.

—JAMES HOWELL

The way that sociologist Arthur Frank has looked at himself and his illness has led to living "actively" with it. "Cancer never disappears," he believes. "I could be having a recurrence now and not yet know it; you can only live in remission."[71] Although "cures" do occur in cancer, I like to remind myself that life itself is a remission, since the death rate for every one of us is 100 percent. We are all terminal cases. So everyone qualifies for the remission society.

Living in or out of remission from illness is most effective and enjoyable when we grow to appreciate fully what we have, regardless of our condition, and explore the opportunities life is present-ing to us in both health and disease. Frank has chosen to live his ill-ness actively, to see it as "just another way of living" and to gain from the possibilities it offers—"closer relationships, more poignant appreciations, clarified values."[72] He says, "You are enti-tled to mourn what you can no longer be, but do not let this mourning obscure your sense of what you can become."[73]

The number of people who find they have gained from their experience of living with pain or a chronic condition is astonish-ing. I kept being surprised by the ways the women in our breast cancer study told me their lives have become better. But before considering how people become better from being severely tested by pain and illness, we need to look more deeply at what their different kind of health means.

Chapter Two

SHIFTING

OUR

IDENTITY

Health is not a condition of matter . . . .
nor can the material senses bear
reliable testimony on the subject of health.

—MARY BAKER EDDY

If I say I am a well person, although a medical assessment shows otherwise, I am talking about having an inner sense of health. Health is something we have at a fundamental level of being, not something we get. We have it despite the storms that may occur in our bodies and lives.[1] We may lose parts or functions of our bodies, but our essence as a person retains its integrity, its health,[2] and is there for us to claim.

When I say I am well inside myself, I am expressing an identity I have that encompasses more than the body. It is a basic identity of wholeness grounded in an order bestowed on us as a natural state.[3]

When people report on clinical surveys that they are well persons—although they have chronic conditions or other physical illness—they are expressing this basic self-identity of health. It is such an identity that gives us a sense of being well inside ourselves. It is there for us to claim although our bodies may be sick and we have recurring pain.[4]

The body provides us with an identity on one level. On another level we have a more basic identity tied to a deeper wholeness and intelligence. Quantum physics recognizes "a profound wholeness in nature . . . a fundamental inseparability of those aspects . . . formerly conceived to be separate."[5] As part of nature, we are part of this wholeness and the self is embedded in a larger web of life.[6] We are joined to a universal energy and order that quantum physicists know as the unified field.[7] The field has coherence and an intelligence that we are part of at the very ground of our being. The physical theory about this deeper level is that it is a universal field of form and flux, pattern and power, comprising the fundamental reality of all that is. It has a dynamic harmony that physicists call intelligent, and it is enmeshed in the larger knowledge that Einstein said transcends human intelligence. If we are religious, we identify this grander knowledge with God.

A DEEPER REALITY

We shall never cease from exploration
And the end of all our exploring
Will be to arrive where we started
And know the place for the first time.

—T. S. ELIOT

When we meditate, pray, lose ourselves in breath-taking beauty, profoundly connect with another person, and otherwise experience transforming moments in our lives, we become aware of the power and presence of this deeper reality. Although we may normally be unaware of our connection to a "perfect health" that our basic identity represents, its order and wholeness is inside us as a natural state, an "inner blueprint that cannot be erased."[8] An underlying principle of the emerging practice of transpersonal medicine is that our ordinary, personal "self" is a "partial manifestation or expression" of a vast field of consciousness, which is our "origin and destination."[9] As expressed in the major religions of the world, we are made in a divine image and retain the inner stamp of God's healing grace. Wordsworth's famous lines tell us that "trailing clouds of glory do we come/From God, who is our home.[10] Our most indelible identity, then, is with a transcendent reality.

Dr. Willis Harman, a Stanford University professor of applied science and engineering, became dissatisfied at age 36 with science's ontological assumption that evolutionary random events, giving rise to molecules and their mechanical motions, explain life. But his true awakening came years later, around age 60, after a profound depression. He said:

> This episode seemed to have to do with the deeper realization—I felt it somewhere in the region of my stomach—that my life was approaching its end. It did feel like a death experience, and then one morning I walked up a hill to see the sunrise and in one indescribable moment all the depression lifted. Life was joyous again.[11]

What Harman came to realize from his hilltop experience is that the only lasting identity is with something greater than the material self. "I am merely a part of the Whole," and "the deepest pleasure in life is serving that Whole."[12] Harman went on to serve many years as president of the Institute of Noetic Sciences and was a highly productive author and lecturer until his death in 1997.

On a health survey, when we report that we are a "healthy" or "fairly healthy" person even though we have a chronic condition, pain, or serious illness, we are drawing upon information from our "inner blueprint" or identity for our self-appraisal. I can be well inside myself; I can be well as a *person* but be dying. In both instances, I am expressing a self-identity that exceeds the body or is other than the physical aspect of my being.

Illness reduces us, makes us feel "smaller," because we hurt and focus on the physical. By identifying with a wholeness larger than the physical, we "increase" the self and expand it beyond the body. We shift our identity to the nonphysical self and hurt less. The Dutch philosopher Spinoza said "love is the increase of self by means of other."[13]

WHAT SOUNDS THROUGH US AT OUR CORE

We are made of star dust, of the cosmos,
of the stuff of where we come from.

—CARL SAGAN

In Latin, the word for "person" is *personare,* meaning "through sound." When we consider the sound of all the words for God or spirit in the languages of the world, most have an "aahh" sound: God, Yahweh, Allah, Brahman, Atman, Jah, Ra, Ram, Baal, Ahara Mazda, Og, Mah.[14] Joachim-Ernst Berendt, a musicologist and writer, observes that "at the basis of the concept of *person* . . . stands a concept of sound: 'through the tone.' If nothing sounds through from the bottom of the being, a human being is human biologically, at best, but is not a *per-son,* because he does not live through the *son* (the tone or sound)."[15] Such an individual, he believes, is not registering "the sound which is the world" or "the Great Tone," which is God. We register the sound when we stay in touch with our essence, which connects us with an incorruptible harmony. In a more literal sense, humans throughout the world, from the beginning of recorded time, have used harps, drums, pipes, flutes, and cymbals to produce sound in healing rituals for the purpose of evoking divine power and recovering wholeness.

Dr. Candace Pert, a neuroscientist at Georgetown University and a former chief of brain chemistry at the National Institutes of Health, notes there is "a theme in all the world's religions" that sounds through people at their innermost level. It is what she calls "the love vibration" and it "is pivotal. It makes us feel better, it's healing, and one day when we have totally worked out the physics of it . . . when we've gone beyond the biochemistry of emotions, there's no doubt that the love vibration's going to be some

fundamental tone and we're going to understand why it's so healing and why it's so good."[16]

BETTER QUALITY OF LIFE

As is a tale, so is life:

not how long it is

but how good it is,

is what matters.

—SENECA

But what good is being well as a person—registering "the Great
Tone"—if our body is sick and in pain? There are several benefits
we can expect. As we saw in Chapter 1, when we believe we are
healthy, despite laboratory tests and a medical assessment showing
otherwise, we are more likely to live longer. A healthy self-rating is
also associated with a better quality of life, an ability to rise above
our pain and see the good in life. Our health belief reflects our
well-being in quite a literal sense. We believe we are well in our
being. Because of whatever infirmity or disability we have, we may
be limited in what we can *do* but not in what we *are*. We are identifying with being well in a sense beyond the body, where our basic
self remains intact and whole.

Naya, Frederick Buechner's maternal grandmother, kept well
connected to her core self, he remembers. "Even when her life was
shattered by the deaths of people she loved and by other kinds of
loss or failure, she remained so serene and intact that it was as if she
lived out of some deep center within herself that was beyond the

reach of circumstance."[17] Two decades later, when Naya was 94 and was "too old and frail with a broken hip" to live anywhere but a nursing home, she wrote Buechner a letter describing herself as "an old crone in a dark little room."[18] But Naya was much more than this. She was "without either bitterness or complaint" and still whole at the core. Buechner, a Presbyterian minister turned writer of fine books, says:

> There was a room inside her which was neither dark nor little, and in that room she continued to be—how to put words to it without tarnishing it?—full of wit and eloquence to the end. It is a glimpse of at least some important aspect of wholeness that I carry with me to this day, a bit of banister to hold onto as I prepare, myself, to climb the dark stair.[19]

WELL IN ONE'S BEING

When I would recreate myself,
I seek the darkest wood. . . .
There is the strength . . . .
—THOREAU

Because basic identity as a person is grounded in a core sense of being, I can be well inside myself even if I am dying, as Naya showed us. When Dr. Balfour Mount trained with Cicely Saunders of London, who started the now-worldwide hospice movement, he learned to ask terminal patients this question: "When were you last well?"[20] A widow in her seventies with metastatic breast cancer whose pain could not be controlled replied, "Do you mean physically?" "No, I mean inside yourself." The woman said, "Doctor, I've never been well a day in my life . . . . I've been sick in mind and spirit every day of my life." Many dying patients, Mount found, were more fortunate. They could die "well," because they held on to a core sense of nonphysical health even when the body experienced illness and pain (see Chapter 10). Mount, a surgical oncologist in Canada who himself had cancer, speaks also of dying "healed."[21] When we die healed, we have used our inner health to bring together what has been split in our lives, in our emotions, in our relationships with others and with God. Living or dying, being well inside ourselves is a matter of tapping the peace and order at the base of our being.[22]

JUST A DELUSION?

But again, is perceiving ourselves as "well" when we are sick just a pollyannish self-delusion? As Idler, who has studied subjective health as much or more than any other researcher, reported, "those who rate their health in positive terms despite the presence of medical problems have been seen as engaging in denial of significant symptoms, or lacking necessary health knowledge, or possessing a poor memory, any of which could lead to the ignoring of serious symptoms and a failure to seek appropriate medical care."[23]

The facts, however, refute such speculations, because studies show that people can be both fully aware of the severity of their physical condition *and* retain a sense of well-being.[24] If our self-rating of being in excellent or good health were so invalid because of any of the possible reasons Idler identifies, then it could not have the positive effect on our future mortality that it has. It is possible to have pain and illness on one level of our being, the physical, and health and wholeness on another, even more basic level of self. So when we hear someone say, "I feel whole despite my illness," we are hearing that person's truth. This was a point made by Virginia Veatch, who directs a cancer help program in Inverness, California, at a Commonweal Conference on New Directions in Health and Healing.[25] Veatch herself, only the year before, had undergone bypass surgery for coronary heart disease, a lumpectomy for breast cancer, and was still on crutches from a broken hip suffered in a fall.

A SELF-IDENTITY OF HEALTH

. . . to remain strong, no matter what shocks come in at the periphery and tend to crack the hub of the wheel.

—ANNE MORROW LINDBERGH

When we make self-evaluations of our health, particularly when we're asked if we see ourselves as a healthy or sick person, we seem to be revealing more about what we perceive our "self-identity" to be than what our physical condition is.[26] This is not to say that how we perceive our health is only a question of believing in wholeness at a core level. The more medical conditions we have and the more severe they are, the more likely we will see ourselves as sick. But many people who have a chronic illness or disorder, such as those in the remission society and pain fellowship, still see themselves as basically well despite lapses or stays in the overt role of a sick person. These individuals are drawing on a deeper sense of self for their health.

In a study of Israelis age 65 and older, in which 70 percent of the 1,112 who were evaluated had at least two diseases and only 10 percent reported none, survival five years later was five times greater among those who said they consider themselves a healthy or fairly healthy person.[27] Dr. Giora Kaplan and his colleagues in the Department of Clinical Epidemiology at Chaima Medical Center, who did the Israeli study, noted that "self-identity...is a more basic and, possibly, more conceptually stable perception than health status," which changes as our physical condition or degree of disability changes.[28]

Sickness, for sure, can have a profound effect on how we look, act, and present ourselves to others. But a self-identity of health goes beyond these. In chronic conditions, depending on how we are feeling and responding to treatment, we may present an image of health at one time and of illness at another. Sociologist Talcott Parsons of Harvard, who studied sick roles, defined them in terms of whether we act sick—go to the doctor, take medicine, lie in bed, become dependent. The more we practice such behavior, the more identified we become with it.[29] In later studies, clinical epidemiologists Stanislav Kasl and Sidney Cobb in 1966 concluded that such behavior leads to an identity as a sick person.[30]

I have looked sick, acted sick, and felt sick many times. On occasion I—meaning all of me—have felt sick in every part of my being, particularly during deep depressions. Only slowly did I discover I had a deeper strength and found ways to access it. By the time I had surgery to remove a large, spreading cluster of basal cell carcinomas in the middle of my chest, I could identify more with being healthy "inside myself" than with being objectively sick or impaired. My basic identity, grounded in a sense of wholeness, told me one thing, and my draining wound and pain something else. The amount of bleeding and the rate of healing that I experienced varied with how well I stayed attached to this fundamental identity. When I got caught up in anxiety about my family, my work, or my writing, the capillaries responsible for building "bridges" between the two sides of my wound and filling in the wide hole with connective tissue, turned pale and stopped doing the repair work. When I reconnected with my inner health, they brightened with good blood and oxygen flow and continued making the tissue connections necessary for healing.

SUBJECTIVELY WELL, OBJECTIVELY SICK

Being defined, then, as either sick or well, depending on how we carry out our roles and how we may feel at a given time, does not fit many of us with chronic or recurring conditions. As we have seen, the prevailing concept of health as the absence of disease or disorder excludes those who see themselves as well or "persevere and succeed in spite of their illness" or pathology.[31] A "person who cannot walk and must move about in a wheelchair can hardly be called 'well'" under the conventional definition of health.[32] Consequently, all of us in such circumstances of pain, illness, or disability have to define ourselves. "The remission society is left to be either a demilitarized zone in between" the kingdoms of sick and well, "or else it is a secret society within the realm of the healthy."[33]

Having a subjective state of health while objectively sick has been a well-kept secret of many remission society members and those with recurrent disease who rate themselves as well people. This self-identity as a healthy person is something not only deeper but wider than our physical status. The self encompasses more than our body, behaviors, feelings, roles, or the impressions we give to others. We have an aspect of self that is undeniably physical, another that is focused on our relationships with others (interpersonal), another that strives to achieve and to be competent, another that is spiritual (transpersonal), and a part that is concerned with our inner conflicts and our unconscious (intrapersonal).[34]

When Anatole Broyard, the well-known literary critic, was suddenly struck with prostate cancer, he wanted his doctors to do more than just scan his body and treat his physical self. "I'd like my doctor to scan *me,* to grope for my spirit as well as my prostate."[35] Otherwise, Broyard was convinced, "I am nothing but my illness."

In my case, I can't be well or whole as a person if I identify only with my body. I have a scarred-over hole 3 inches in diameter in the middle of my chest from surgery. Women treated for breast cancer have holes in their breasts, if they have any breasts at all. They are not less whole because their bodies are. I am not less whole.

BUTCH AND PHINEAS GAGE

But because we are embodied creatures with self-images that draw heavily on our physical intactness, damage to the body can change how we look at ourselves and feel about our lives.[36] We had a tragic "identity" case at the Texas Medical Center, where my school, the University of Texas School of Public Health, is located. It involved a 35-year-old patient named "Butch," who had been burned over 96 percent of his body yet miraculously survived. His nose was burned off, his ears were gone, very little was left to identify him. Skin grafts were taken and harvested from the base of his scrotum and the soles of his feet. He was on a ventilator, he had severe nutritional problems and infections, he had kidney damage. Yet his will to live and modern technology saved him.

Then one day, six months later, Butch accidently saw himself in a mirror. He was horrified. He couldn't believe what he saw. Twelve days later, Butch died. Dr. Rebecca Clearman, his chief physician at The Texas Rehabilitation and Research Institute, reported: "Nothing was wrong. He wasn't infected. His heart, lungs, and internal organs were working perfectly. There wasn't a medication side effect. There simply was no reason. The coroner said it was a 'voluntary suicide,'" meaning he died from giving up his will to live.[37]

Butch was burned so severely in his body and was so traumatized by the look in the mirror that he could not access his core sense of self, his "remembered wellness." Our primary identity is captured in the memory cells and deep structures of the brain that give us a sense of self. These neurons and circuits extend from the amygdala deep in the brain to the frontal cortex at the top. This core contains the deepest and most enduring layers of our personality.[38] The most compelling evidence for this neural self and identity dates back more than 150 years.

A man named Phineas Gage lost his sense of self, his identity, and made history in the annals of medicine and neurology. In a freak accident, on September 13, 1848, in Vermont, a long, iron bar was driven through Gage's face, skull, brain, and beyond by an explosion on the railroad track construction site where he was a foreman. Stunned only momentarily, Gage, 25, regained full consciousness and "was able to talk and even walk with the help of his men."[39] The iron bar landed some distance away. Although Gage survived and fully recovered physically, he became a different person. He had been "responsible, intelligent, and socially well-adapted...a favorite with his peers and elders."[40] Now he was irresponsible, profane, offensive toward others, and uncaring. His employers, who had deemed him "the most efficient and capable man" they had, finally let him go. His friends and acquaintances said, "Gage is no longer Gage." He had lost his identity. Gage died 12 years later in San Francisco, never having regained his sense of self or the identity he once had. No autopsy was performed, but after his burial, his family consented to having the body exhumed so his skull could be studied by medical researchers. Damage involved both left and right portions of his prefrontal cortex.

Remembering Wholeness

This is the great error of our day in the treatment of the human being, that the physicians separate the soul from the body.

—PLATO

As long as the prefrontal cortex structures remain intact and we have a mind and brain capable of presenting a "full picture of the body and the world around it," we can reclaim our natural state of wholeness.[41] The evidence that such a natural state exists comes from different lines of inquiry. For instance, when people suffer pain from "phantom limbs"—limbs that have been amputated—the brain remembers a "wholeness" and registers pain where once there was a leg.[42]

We are "wired"—have neuronal patterns laid down in our brains—for wholeness, for connections not only to our bodily parts but to other people and the universe in which we live. When we truly connect with another person or when we meditate, pray, or hear music that moves us, we often experience a unity, a oneness that is a source of strength and identity. Poets, philosophers, theologians, and practitioners of Eastern medicine have long described that source as constituting our core identity, our inner health, our essence, our spirit and soul.

Even when the brain has been damaged by disease, some patients, long immobilized by encephalitis or Parkinsonism, can draw on their essence, this source of "remembered wellness," and temporarily move their bodies freely again when they hear music that stirs them.[43] Neurologist Oliver Sachs has written about one "frozen" post-encephalitic patient, once a music teacher, who "said she had been 'demusicked' by her disease."[44] But "she would suddenly recover herself, albeit briefly, if she was 'remusicked' again ('You are the music/while the music lasts'—T. S. Eliot[45])." Whenever we truly lose ourselves in something larger, we are on the path for reclaiming our essence, our inner health.

Jimmie, another of Sachs' patients, had such severe neurological damage that he could not "remember isolated items for more than a few seconds" and had "dense amnesia."[46] But "humanly, spiritually," Jimmie at times would stop being "restless, bored, and lost" and become "deeply attentive to the beauty and soul of the world...the aesthetic, the moral, the religious, the dramatic....Empirical science...takes no account of the soul, no account of what constitutes and determines personal being." Sachs makes the point that:

> Perhaps there is a philosophical as well as a clinical lesson here: that in Korsakov's or dementia, other such catastrophes, however great the organic damage...there remains the undiminished possibility of reintegration by art, by communion, by touching the human spirit, and this can be preserved in what seems at first a hopeless state of neurological devastation.[47]

LIFTING BEYOND PAIN

Pain and pleasure, like light and darkness, succeed each other.

—LAURENCE STERNE

If we have a passion for a goal, an activity, an idea, a place, a person, God, we can often lift ourselves beyond chronic pain and the misery of a disorder (see Chapters 5 and 6). I have a passion for mountains, and years ago discovered that I stopped hurting when I began my ascent to a summit, captured by the beauty of changing fauna, flora, and sky all the way up. Chronic pain specialists know much more now than in previous years about managing the relentless hurting the brain registers from a bad back, belly, elbow, knee, or some other part. When we become engrossed in a passion and get out of ourselves, we suffer less because we have something better to do, which confirms a principle now known in the pain literature as "Fordyce's Law," after Dr. Wilbert Fordyce of the University of Washington Medical School, a pioneer in pain research.[48] We tap into a deeper source of wholeness, a different kind of health.

To become immersed in a passion, we must have a caring center. Gage not only lost a self-identity but his capacity for caring. There have been a number of Phineas Gages since the first one. Dr. Antonio R. Damasio, professor of neurology at the University of Iowa Medical College, has studied more than 12 patients with damage to frontal lobes, either from injury or surgery to remove a tumor. All showed a "decision-making defect and flat emotion and feeling."[49]

CARING IS PRIMARY

Life comes from physical survival, but the good life comes from what we care about.

—ROLLO MAY

If we have an "affective indifference" toward life, whether from brain damage or some other cause, we lack the caring required to invest so strongly in something that we are lifted out of ourselves. But, again, even in a few cases of frontal lobe damage, a temporary reconnecting with a core caring center, beyond the ravages of disordered physiology, has been reported. "Another patient of mine," Sachs said, "had massive front lobe damage, rendering him completely 'flat' emotionally, seemingly incapable of any normal feeling. But he loved music (country music especially), and when he sang, as he sometimes did spontaneously, he would come alive in the most remarkable way, as if the music could give him, transiently, what his cortex had lost."[50]

The caring center is primary, Dr. Patricia Benner of the University of California, San Francisco, has noted.[51] As long as the caring structure is intact, we can access what it takes for a sense of wholeness and health that remains with us in the presence of physical disorder and disease. Caring is what connects us to the world beyond self and heals us. In a very physiological way, caring has beneficial effects. For instance, in a well-controlled study, a group of individuals who spent five minutes experiencing feelings of care and compassion produced a significant increase in levels of S–IgA, antibodies that provide a first-line defense against germs in the upper respiratory tract, gastrointestinal system, and urinary tract.[52] In contrast, persons in the experiment who induced feelings of anger and frustration did not raise their IgA levels. For them the antibodies remained low for five hours, while in the care and compassion group the increase of IgA persisted for an hour.

Caring that connects us is different from anxious, neurotic caring, which expresses itself in excessive concern about what people think of us, say about us, in obsessing about being important, making a name, accumulating power and possessions. Self-based or ego-based caring separates us from warmth and love in relationships while self-less caring—ego-free—joins us to larger wholes.[53]

Many in the remission society and fellowship of pain have moved toward ego-free caring. That is part of the experience of improving as a person, which many see as how they have benefited from their illness.

Chapter Three

IMPROVING

AS A

PERSON

There is a piece of fortune in misfortune.

—JAPANESE PROVERB

Wₕhat we can become from our experience of recurring illness is a better person. A frequent finding in studies of people with chronic conditions and those surviving life-threatening disease is the conviction that "I am stronger now" or "I am braver" or "I have been tested and didn't fall to pieces" or "I see more now" or "I'm just a better person."[1]

Although people who give such reports also acknowledge that "they may not have chosen their circumstances, in many ways they are glad the event happened; this is true even in cases involving permanent disability."[2] Some even say that their cancer or their heart disease or their injury was "the best thing that has happened" to them. In my interviews, I asked 13 women from our pilot project the question of whether there was any value or benefit that they believed they had found in having cancer. Twelve answered yes. Most said, in effect, they had become a better person.

Those who are convinced they have benefited by their trauma tell of being more patient, more understanding, more compassionate, more "awake," and more appreciative of how good life is.[3] Max Lerner, who spoke from experiencing both cancer and two heart attacks, said: "My illness gave the idea of the sacral in my life a depth it lacked.... I find all sorts of things now—even 'profane' things—to be sacred. Our few acres of grass and trees at White Hedges, whether morning, dusk, or full moon—I get a shiver of delight from gazing at them."[4]

A WAKE-UP CALL AND PATIENCE

Adopt the pace of nature;

her secret is patience.

—EMERSON

In a recent cancer study, questionnaires were mailed to several thousand women on the East and West Coasts who were diagnosed with breast cancer up to five years earlier, and 800 chose to write in blank space on the form about how cancer had changed their lives.[5] A large majority cited benefits from their illness, such as "it has made me appreciate life more" or "it gave my life a purpose" or "it was a wake-up call for me." As one cancer survivor in England put it: "Yes, for me cancer was most certainly a wake-up call, an opportunity to heal and evolve through the illness."[6] Another research team found that more than 90 percent of the cancer patients they studied "reported positive changes in their lives as a result of the cancer experience."[7]

Many of those who said they appreciate life more also mentioned they have learned to be more patient. Patience rewards us in science as well as healing. Nobel laureate Barbara McClintock made plain that she couldn't do her work with plants, with the genes she studied in corn, without "holding communion" with them, and having the patience to start with a seedling and watch it slowly grow.[8] She also had the patience to see the myriad subtleties that give flowers their personality. "In the summertime," she said, "when you walk down the road, you'll see the tulip leaves, if it's a little warm, turn themselves around so their backs are toward the sun. You can just see where the sun hits them and where the sun doesn't hit . . . they move around a great deal" and "are fantastically beyond our wildest expectations."[9]

EMERGENCE OF THE TRUE SELF

In a study that included AIDS as well as cancer patients, "many...believed that their diagnoses had been blessings in many ways" and had changed their lives for the better.[10] Findings from a study that focused on 25 women, age 40 to 78, who had survived breast cancer for at least five years without recurrence, showed that many reported the "emergence of a more authentic self as a result of the cancer experience."[11] They "emerged...with a clearer sense of self, gratitude for life, and strength and confidence in their ability to manage life crises."[12]

One woman experienced personal growth by "healing the wounds of growing up in an alcoholic family."[13] She became closer to her husband and friends and placed value on "being real" and "no longer a phoney." Such changes often occur after we learn to deal better with the fear that comes with life-threatening illness and trauma. "Fear prevents us from distinguishing our true identity from our persona."[14]

Our true identity, as distinguished from the face we often present to the world, is embedded in a deeper reality that extends beyond persona. It is the base from which we bond with others and our God. It is a base of unity. We often discover this unity by being severely tested by pain, by threat of death, by a wrenching loss. None of us wants to face such tests, but if, by chance, we sail through life without being tested, we sense we have missed something important and don't know what we are made of.

WHAT BEING SEVERELY TESTED REVEALS

Gerald Coffee, an art major in college, spent seven years and nine days in a North Vietnamese prisoner-of-war camp after his Navy plane was hit by antiaircraft fire.[15] He endured torture, a broken arm that wasn't set for weeks, and long solitary confinement until his captors ran out of space at Hoa Lo and had to house the prisoners in proximity to one another. The Americans perfected an elaborate communication system by tapping codes on their cell walls and not only kept each other's spirits up but even engaged in a debate as to whether an engineer or a liberal arts major was best equipped to survive such harsh conditions. Powerful bonding developed. "Our motto," Coffee said, "was Unity over Self."[16]

When Gerry Coffee gives talks in the United States, people sometimes come up to him and confess "a stab of envy for an experience that had stripped him to the core of his being yet revealed hidden strengths." Coffee is not surprised. "What they're talking about is a rite of passage, something that forces you to discover yourself, your connection to other people, your relationship to spirituality. Anything that helps us do that is conducive to survival."[17]

HEALTHIER FROM DISEASE

And makes us rather bear those ills we have
Than fly to others that we know not of?
—SHAKESPEARE

Chronic disability or disease, no matter whether we have it or one of our children or other family member does, not only can bring us closer to others but can also teach us what is important in life and lead us to discovering a core health and deep strength we didn't know we had. These are the benefits we may receive if we choose to look for the positive contributions that pain or impairment makes to our lives rather than to focus only on the physical costs we bear.[18]

If our life has gone off track and we have lost a sense of direction, it may take a life-threatening diagnosis and illness to "provide a kind of shock" that forces us to face our own mortality and re-think our priorities.[19] From such an experience we can emerge happier and more at peace with ourselves. We also can become healthier from disease. A finding from the AIDS and cancer patients study cited earlier was that a number "felt they had become healthier as a result of having their diagnosis," Dr. Patricia Fryback of the University of Southern Mississippi reported.[20] At the heart of experiencing health in disease is an enlarged awareness of ourselves and our lives, an expanded consciousness. A polio survivor puts it this way:

> Far away from the hospital experience, I can evaluate what I have learned.... I know my awareness of people has deepened and increased, that those who are close to me can want me to turn all my heart and mind and attention to their problems. I could not have learned *that* dashing all over the tennis court."[21]

How Can Cancer Be a "Blessing"?

What we count the ills of life

are often blessings in disguise,

resulting in good to us in the end.

—MATTHEW HENRY

Whatever benefits we receive, they are often a turning point in our lives. One of the women in our cancer study who told me that "cancer has been a blessing" for her explained that it led to an awakening for her and her family, one that changed the way they were living.[22] Anna is convinced, as are most of the other women interviewed, that stress and cancer are related. She said her life had been very stressful for at least five years before her diagnosis because of many moves due to frequent transfers of her husband to different cities in the United States and South America, because of the death of his mother from breast cancer and—also important, in Anna's judgment—because of the high-fat diet she and her family ate and their faulty nutrition. She sees the shock of getting cancer as a turning point that led her to a study of stress and nutrition, which resulted in the family's changing their lifestyle and eating habits.

Calling cancer "a blessing" or "the best thing that ever happened to me" struck Dr. Larry Dossey as "absurd" when he was a young physician.[23] That disease could lead "to an increase in wisdom and understanding, and held lessons that paradoxically made life better" was antithetical to what he had been taught as a clinical scientist. "I was not impressed. Humans will stop at nothing, I told myself, to rationalize their plight."[24] Only after he learned that all of us have a need to find meaning and an explanation when we are struck by a serious illness did Dossey recognize the "wisdom and insight" of people who discover value in trauma and pain and benefit by doing so.[25]

BEST THING THAT EVER HAPPENED?

Perceiving benefit in a calamity is an attitude that those who have never had such experiences often find hard to understand. A man in his 30s was being interviewed by a television show host about the accident he had when he was 17 and dived into a shallow pool. He ended up with a broken neck and a paralysis that affects much of his body, including both legs.[26] The man told his interviewer: "This is the best thing that ever happened to me." More than incredulous, she replied: "Oh, yeah, come on, that's ridiculous."[27]

The man went on to explain that at 17, "I was in a beery fog. I never thought about anything except drinking and fooling around with women, and I really didn't make use of anything above my neck." After the accident, he married, had four children, and went on to become the secretary of the British Association of the Disabled. He discovered much value in what was above his neck.[28]

Parents who have children disabled from birth also cope more successfully when they choose to see benefits in their experience. Their children do better too. Research shows that "the comparatively few mothers who were unable to find any benefits had children who developed less optimally during their second year of life."[29]

Parents who construe benefits take pride in what the child can do rather than dwell on the child's deficiencies. They report a personal strength and family closeness they didn't have before and come to see that "persons with disabilities enrich the quality of life for family and friends."[30]

"CLARIFIED MY VALUES"

Nobody sees a flower really —
it is so small—we haven't time
—and to see takes time. Like to
have a friend takes time.

—GEORGIA O'KEEFE

What Robert Eliot discovered was a benefit of a different kind. A hard-driving academic physician, his ambition was to be chief of cardiology at a major medical school by age 40.

He didn't realize his ambition until age 43, at the University of Nebraska, so "all I had to do was run a little faster and I'd be back on track."[31] At age 44, he suffered a heart attack.

> During three months of recuperation, I rethought my life and clarified my values. As Nietzsche has observed, 'If you stare long enough into the abyss, it begins to stare back.' I had stared into the abyss of death and it made me a believer in life.[32]

Eliot also "rediscovered" his wife and family. Years later she told him: "You know, Bob, if you had died from your heart attack, I don't think the kids and I would have missed you. We never really knew you. If you were to die now, we would miss you very much."[33]

Studies show that actual physical gains can be derived from construing value in traumatic experience. Drs. Glenn Affleck and Howard Tennen, in studying survivors of myocardial infarctions discovered that "men who had found benefits soon after their heart attacks were significantly less likely to have another attack in the ensuing eight years, regardless of the severity of their attack."[34]

LEARNING TO RECEIVE AS WELL AS GIVE

Love gives naught but itself
and takes naught but from itself.
Love possesses not nor would be possessed;
For love is sufficient until love.

—KAHLIL GIBRAN

Learning how to receive love was what Dr. Frank Lawlis' heart at-tack taught him.[35] For most of his life he had taken care of people and had many who loved him. But receiving their love had been difficult. Long before he became a psychologist, he took on the caring role for others. His father died when he was 19, and he in-herited the job of advising, supporting, and helping friends and rel-atives. Much of his career as a psychologist has been on the giving end of empathy, love, and compassion. His heart attack brought him "hundreds of calls, cards, and gifts, and each one touched me in a specific and wonderful way."[36] For the first time, he was ac-cepting of all the love and didn't feel he should be giving it and not receiving it.

In an epilogue to his book on *Transpersonal Medicine: A New Ap-proach to Healing Body-Mind-Spirit*, Lawlis wrote: "I am grateful for this experience, and I can better understand why other cultures so respect a survivor. Through trauma and disease we learn so much about ourselves, tapping a vital source of courage in order to cope. This disease has touched me at multiple levels, and I imagine that more lessons await me."[37] One of the underlying principles of transpersonal psychology, which Lawlis has helped pioneer, is that disease and pain present us with an opportunity for personal growth and transformation, which is another way of saying that good can come out of bad.

STANDING UP TO ANYTHING

. . . I give you my hand!
I give you my love more precious than money . . .
Will you give me yourself? . . .
Shall we stick by each other as long as we live?
—WHITMAN

In both acute life-threatening illness and chronic disorders, such as a congenital disability of a newborn baby, we are confronted with existential issues out of which to mine something of value. A parent of a severely disabled child, whose life began in crisis in the newborn intensive care unit, describes the experience this way:

> The good that came out of this was how we reacted as a couple. Something like this could tear a marriage apart . . . but instead it has brought us closer. Right after she was born, I remember this revelation. She was teaching us something . . . how to keep things in perspective . . . to realize what's important. I've learned that everything is tentative and that you never know what life will bring. I've learned that I'm a much stronger person than I had thought. I look back, see how far I've come, and feel very pleased. The good that's come from this is that I marvel what a miracle she is . . . what a miracle that she's alive and that we are going to take her home.[38]

Dana, 45, another woman in our breast cancer project, told me she discovered similar value and benefit in having faced her serious illness.[39] "I found I had an inner strength and can stand up to any-thing." She has found more patience, understanding, and empathy as qualities coming out of her experience with cancer and a radical mastectomy. "It has also prepared me better for my own dying, whenever that comes."

The feeling that "I can stand up to anything" takes confidence. Where does that confidence come from? Certainly being tested and not falling to pieces is part of it. A sense of competence also plays a role. But a deeper part of confidence is nurtured by a feeling of being loved (see Chapter 9 on resilience). For instance, in a study of 135 multiple sclerosis patients, love was found to be "the most powerful predictor of self-esteem," which, in turn, had the strongest influence over coping successfully with the disease.[40]

COURAGE BUILDS ON COURAGE, LOVE ON LOVE

But when two people are one in their inmost hearts,
They shatter even the strength of iron or of bronze.
—I CHING

From adversity, we can also learn courage and love and how each builds on the other as we cope with threats to our physical health and life. Both courage and love help us discover our inner sense of health, which releases an energy and strength we didn't have be-fore. Spouses and other family members can be inspired and made stronger by one who is sick and shows increasing love and forti-tude. "Some kind of energy... can be transferred among individu-als," an energy that moves us toward wholeness.[41]

A powerful source of this energy comes from the principle of mutuality, which says that when we truly connect with others, when we respond to life with openness and receptivity, we vitalize ourselves and those around us.[42] The psychological and physical truth in the principle of mutuality was recognized by Shakespeare when he referred to those human responses—"virtues"—which "shining upon others heat them and they retort that heat again to the first giver."[43] Courage builds on courage, love on love.

Dr. Sol Cohen, whose physician wife shared a practice of medicine with him for many years, said he felt "ennobled" by how she dealt with her long episode of breast cancer, which ended in her death. They kept building on each other's greater courage and love "until I really felt we had touched God."[44] "I became a better human being, a better doctor," he said.

PERCEIVING BENEFITS IS NOT DENYING THE PAIN

Because advantage from adversity does strike many as contradictory, we must ask, as Affleck and Tennen did: "Are parents who find the 'silver lining' in what many would view as a personal tragedy turning away from reality? Are they 'denying' the painful truths of this traumatic experience?"[45] In answer, they cite research showing that "parents who find more benefits from this situation are no more or less likely than parents finding fewer benefits to endorse statements about the harmful aspects of this experience."[46] The conclusion is that "perceiving benefits does not imply denial of threat."[47]

Similarly, studies of both cancer and AIDS have shown that those who cope best see value in their experience with illness but not to the exclusion of recognizing negative effects and the threat to life.[48] If perceiving benefit means having some "positive illusions," as Taylor calls them, then the evidence is that we are better off with them than without them.[49]

Denial of a threatening reality is detrimental when it keeps us from exploring and considering what value there may be in the painful, negative circumstance we are stuck with. It constitutes false hope, hope that does not acknowledge the darkness we are in.[50] After some initial struggling, most people who suffer serious setbacks reach the point where "one's circumstances are not disavowed" and there is a "focus on possible positive outcomes and positive aspects of one's situation."[51]

As we noted in Chapter 1, our subjective sense of health, our belief in our own capacity to experience life as good in the face of trauma and tragedy, has profound influence on our physical functioning and feeling. Health, both inner and outer, both subjective and objective, has to do with well-being, which we enhance when we find love, meaning, mastery, or a sense of coherence in whatever condition or circumstance life presents to us.

WHOLE WHEN OUR BODY IS NOT

The whole is more than the sum of the parts.
—ARISTOTLE

Experiencing ourselves as well in our being comes from making our life whole even when our body is not. What does "whole" mean in terms of what we experience in our lives and inside ourselves?

> To feel whole is to feel 'at one' and undivided; it is to experience, at least for a moment, a unity and harmony with life. It is to feel at peace with ourselves and others, and to have a sense of our place in

the larger scheme of things. This experience of unity affirms that life is worth living and that loneliness, grief, and other heartaches can be transcended.[52]

How whole our life is, then, depends on the quality of our relationships—interiorly, with each aspect of the self (mind, body, spirit), and exteriorly, with our work, our family, friends, neighbors, and community. On a different dimension is the relationship we have with a transcendent reality, which is not only God[53] but also the reality we experience when the beauty of nature, music, art, or poetry takes us out of ourselves, or the love of country or service lifts us beyond our egos. When we transcend, we rise above our limitations, physical or psychological, and bond with something larger than self, larger than our problem.

A relationship with the transcendent is as vital to keeping the self whole and healthy as is satisfying interpersonal and achievement needs. The 40 scholars who wrote the massive *Columbia History of the World* concluded that there is a "call to transcendence that the human spirit requires."[54] Dr. Ellen Idler of Rutgers University (see Chapter 1), who has extensively studied subjective health among the sick and impaired, has found that cultivating a spiritual sense of self is associated with better health and less disability.[55]

To the extent that we feel a part of others, a part of the world around us, and part of a larger reality, studies suggest we will experience a sense of wholeness. For Arthur Frank, "Seeing the world from a bed in the cancer ward is like seeing it from outer space; it is rather small and fundamentally whole. To be ill, to share in the suffering of being human is to know your place in that whole, to know your connection with others."[56] Serious illness and impending death can bring out the deepest, most authentic parts of us, parts we may have kept under wraps because we thought they did not fit the image of what we "should" be. Often we discover a bonding with others that we didn't know was possible, a deeper and larger connection to the world itself.

To the extent, then, that we derive satisfaction from aspects of our life that are outside the bodily threats of illness or a chronic condition, we will experience a health that "offsets the losses and blows" experienced in the physical area.[57] A fundamental sense of well-being characterizes this kind of health, and well-being is more than the state of the body. Wholeness or well-being may or may not correlate with having a healthy body. As Frank reports: "In the best moments of my illnesses, I have been most whole. In the worst moments of my health I have been sick."[58]

A SENSE OF BEING CONNECTED

. . . We feel we are greater than we know.
—WORDSWORTH

When we have a "connexional experience"—that is, a sense of "binding together parts to form a whole"—we may know it by "a peculiar physical sensation, such as a chill, gooseflesh, or flushing."[59] The experience may be "followed by a lingering feeling of love . . . and a humble feeling that one is part of something bigger than oneself. Such experiences may feel somehow universal and enlarging."[60] There is a sensation of wholeness, a sense of being connected at a core level.

In science and medicine, such descriptions are considered too "soft" and abstruse to be of help in such things as boosting immune function, unclogging arteries, saving kidneys, or transplanting livers. Yet the "connexional experience" is widely enough recognized by clinicians in their encounters with patients that the *Annals of Internal Medicine* published a paper on the subject by Drs. Anthony Suchman of the University of Rochester Medical School and Dale Matthews of the University of Connecticut Department of Medicine. Suchman and Matthews hold that there is within each of us "a sense of isolation, which seems to be an unavoidable consequence of learning to distinguish 'self' from 'other.' "[61] Out of this experience of being separate "arises a drive to reach beyond the boundaries of the self, to feel connected once again to other people and to the world." They believe this sense of belonging in the world brings a sense of meaning. "The need for connection and meaning often goes unrecognized within modern Western culture, yet it remains a need in every person nonetheless. It is through connexional experience that these needs are satisfied."[62] In satisfying them, we gain well-being and an improved quality of life.

But to feel well inside ourselves, we must first overcome not only isolation but fear. Since being whole means acknowledging all parts of who we are, "bitter and sweet, strong and weak," we are called to confront fear directly.[63]

Katie did that. She coped effectively with not only a diagnosis of breast cancer at 29 but surgery and chemotherapy while pregnant with her first child.[64] From such an experience, she emerged as a more open person, more grateful and stronger (see Chapter 9). Her baby daughter was born healthy and continues to show no signs of ill effect from the chemotherapy Katie received. Katie describes her own health as good, good enough for horseback riding and camping out with her husband and now 3-year-old daughter.

PAIN AND JOY SIDE BY SIDE

To remain whole, be twisted.
To become straight, let yourself be bent.
To become full, be hollow.
Be tattered, that you may be renewed.

—*TAO TE CHING*

When well-being becomes the focus of health, then the line between "inner" health and "outer" health—the kind physicians look
for in us—fades. We can be well in our being while impaired physically. As we will see, studies show that chronically ill or disabled
persons have about the same level of well-being as those physically
healthy. Although health as meaning being well inside ourselves,
being undivided and at peace with self and others, is only beginning to be acknowledged, even in the medical literature, we can
find an occasional change in the way health is defined. As one
group of clinical researchers put it: "Health is . . . something positive, a joyful attitude toward life, and a cheerful acceptance of the
responsibilities that life puts upon an individual."[65]

Dr. Viktor Frankl, who survived Auschwitz and Dachau because of his attitude toward life, said that "every situation implies a
call, a responsibility. To this call we must react according to our best
ability and our best conscience. During the three years I spent in
Auschwitz and Dachau I decided that I was responsible for making
use of the slightest chance of survival and ignoring the great danger around me."[66]

Is it possible to be joyful toward life and cheerful about the responsibilities life imposes when our body seems to be failing us

and pain is our most constant companion? If, as research suggests, we can find satisfaction in life without being physically whole and perceive benefits from painful experience, then it is only a short step to peace and joy. Westerners have tended to see this point of view as wishful thinking, as wearing a false smile when despair is more consistent with the painful reality of disease and disorder. In the East, where suffering is considered endemic to life, Buddhists find no paradox in experiencing pain and joy side by side.[67] The Buddhist monks I have met through the yoga practice that my wife and I maintain have been gentle, smiling people. Some of them have undergone great dislocation and distress from the Chinese invasion of Tibet and the trashing of Buddhist temples. Yet they can still dance and sing with joy.

LIVING AND DYING SIMULTANEOUSLY

For me, finding that peace and joy can exist as companions to pain and grief has come partly from the experience of living with the slow, inevitable death of our younger daughter, Elizabeth, and from the realization that "we are all living and dying simultaneously."[68] The last time I was depressed, I began my journey back to feeling alive by attending a seminar on death by a professor of surgery who, unlike most of his colleagues, spends time with his terminal patients, answering questions about dying, and celebrating with them what has been good in their lives. In preparation for our daughter's death, Rita and I began hospice volunteer training at the Texas Medical Center. I became more willing to face death, my own and Elizabeth's, which came the next year. I gradually accepted that "death is lodged in our bowels from the very beginning."[69] I found, as Dr. Herman Feifel kept telling his fellow psychologists for years, that "energies now bound up in continuing strivings to shelve and subdue the idea of death" become available to us, "fortifying our gift for creative splendor against our genius for destruction."[70] In all our "little deaths," we have an opportunity to "glimpse through death's door"[71] that there is not a single way to make life whole and full, that health is as much inner as outer, and that order and satisfaction can be experienced inside in the midst of chaos and disorder outside.

A Sense of Coherence

Wholeness and satisfaction start with a sense of order in our consciousness. For all living organisms, disorder and entropy are "*the* prototypical characteristic."[72] When disease, chronic illness, and pain occur, the disorder is compounded. The ability to keep order in our consciousness, regardless of the trauma we experience, comes from what Dr. Aaron Antonovsky, the longtime, noted medical sociologist in Israel, identified as a sense of coherence—which is a way of perceiving ourselves and the world as having a basic lawfulness and meaningfulness.[73]

Studies confirm that those who score high in coherence cope "amazingly well" when trauma persists.[74] My own experience in doing research with cancer patients and working with others who are faced with recurring, painful physical illness is that those who stay well have a strong sense of coherence. They stay on healthy terms with life and find good in it, although their bodies are hurting or failing.

TURNING "DROSS INTO GOLD"

We were chaff, now we are wheat;

we were dross, now we are gold . . . .

—JAMES BISSE

Health has much to do with how we adapt and respond to what life presents us. The Grant Study has tracked the health of 204 men from the time they were Harvard College sophomores in the early 1940s until the present.[75] Dr. George Vaillant, who has been one of the directors of the research, says that health is best demonstrated when the "going gets tough," when we are faced with the painful reality of serious losses, failures, illness, deaths, and broken dreams. How we respond profoundly affects our physical health status, his research shows.

Across a half century of follow-up, those still surviving and in the best physical and psychological health suffered as many set-backs and losses as the others but adapted by the alchemist's formula of turning "dross into gold."[76] They transformed adversity so that some benefit came out of it, not only to themselves in terms of longevity and quality of life but also to others they reached out to, assisted, and served.[77]

I know two women who became alchemists in the sense Vaillant found among the healthiest in the Grant Study. Both became poets. One, Vassar Miller, lives in Houston, my hometown, and has suffered since birth from cerebral palsy, which impairs her ability to walk, talk, hold a knife or fork, or keep her head from jerking. We have had her meet with University of Texas and Baylor medical students and faculty at the Texas Medical Center and to show slides of her poems, which have been nationally published. I asked her once what "healing" meant to her, and she replied: "freedom from pain." Ms. Miller has lived few days of her life without pain, but her response to these hard terms has been poetry, which has enriched the lives of others as well as her own.

The second woman was Jane Hess Merchant, who had a brittle bone disease called osteogenesis imperfecta and was confined to bed from age 12 until she died 41 years later. By the time she was 23, she was almost totally deaf and nearly blind. Yet she wrote 2,000 poems. When she looked at the world, she saw beyond her own pain and disability and wrote about its beauty and order and the grace of God. Her different kind of health was nourished by a sense of faith and coherence. She knew that discovery of inner health is not a one-time affair but a daily practice. She wrote: "If for one day/I can forget/The nagging care/The needless fret/If for one day/I can believe in life, and joyously/ Receive/The blessings that/Are always mine/Of earth and air/And love divine.... then at last... I may/Learn how to do it/Every day."[78]

KNOWING WHAT MATTERS

Dr. David Myers, a social psychologist at Hope College who knows about disability from inside his own family, has reported on research showing that "the emotional well-being of cancer patients and their satisfaction with different aspects of their lives rivals that of healthy people. People who become blind or paralyzed will, after a period of adjustment, typically recover a near-normal level of day-to-day happiness."[79] Myers' brother Jim is an example. He has a motor neuron disease known as ALS or Lou Gehrig's disease. "Jim has difficulty tying his shoes, buttoning his shirts, typing at his job as a network TV station promotions director."[80] But he has a resilient spirit, takes joy in being with his young daughters, and feels enthusiasm for his volunteer church work. "After staring death in the face, he knows what matters," Myers observes. Jim says: "Life itself seems more precious and real."[81]

Being of service to others, as Jim Myers has been, brings special satisfaction to the wounded well, who want to give help as well as receive it. Dana, the woman who found inner strength in surviving breast cancer, enjoys pairing up with newly diagnosed patients and dispelling some of their fears by conveying her own experience and hopeful outlook. "It makes me feel good to do this and I believe it really does help them," she said.

Some of the first findings on the robustness of persons with life-threatening diseases and chronic conditions came from Dr. Shelley Taylor, a UCLA psychologist who has widely studied patients with cancer and other serious illnesses.[82] She has been struck by the "remarkable" ability of humans to adjust to extremely adverse, "altered life circumstances."[83] Not everyone does adjust, of course, but the majority, after struggling with the damage they have experienced, alter the pain in their bodies by finding value in other areas of their lives. As to the ability of cancer patients, in particular, to find satisfaction and joy, two studies have reported higher quality of life for them than among non-ill comparison samples.[84] Similar findings have been reported for disabled persons.

ON BEING AN ALCHEMIST

By happy alchemy of mind
They turn to pleasure all they find.

—MATTHEW GREEN

Bonnie found much to value and to do in her life although her body was visibly incomplete from birth.[85] She had been born with legs but without arms. She learned to play the organ with her feet, to wash dishes ("I get dishpan feet"), to dress herself ("It's easier for me, I think, than a lot of women"), to drive a car, and to raise two children. Her husband, with whom she corresponded for more than a year before they met and married three months later, said, "I saw a rich philosophy in her." Bonnie never saw her life as not being whole and full. She never considered herself damaged, only different. "All of our lives we strive to be different in what we do, what we look like. And here it was just handed to me on a silver platter: I'm different." Bonnie travelled around the country giving talks about her experience to groups of disabled people. She learned early how to be a successful alchemist.

Alice Stewart Trillin, a former English teacher and mother of two daughters, had lung cancer at age 38 and underwent a lobectomy, chemotherapy, and immunotherapy. She told of her experience in a talk given to students at Cornell and Albert Einstein Medical Schools.[86] "It astonishes me that having faced the terror, we continue to live, even to live with a great deal of joy. It is commonplace for people who have cancer—particularly those who feel as well as I do—to talk about how much richer their lives are because they have confronted death. Yes, my life is very rich."[87]

Lilly, age 52, a woman in our study who suffered recurrence soon afterward with metastases to bones throughout the body, told me that in one sense, "My experience with cancer is the best thing that has ever happened to me."[88] The "kindness and generosity of spirit" she has encountered among both patients and people willing to help has left a lasting impression with her and profoundly affected her outlook on life. (For more on Lilly, see Chapter 4).

The Vassar Millers, Jane Merchants, Jim Myerses, Alice Trillins, Bonnies, Danas, Annas, Katies, Lillys, and Arthur Franks discovered they have a different kind of health, which keeps them well though wounded. This kind of health derives from a basic identity of being whole, which all of us are but few of us recognize. Once we discover what we are at the deepest level of self, we find our inner health.

Chapter Four

DISCOVERING

A NEW KIND

OF HEALTH

The best thing that we're
put here for's to see . . .

—ROBERT FROST

B eing well in the self starts with expanding our consciousness, our way of seeing and understanding. A life-threatening illness may lead us to see and understand that there is a different kind of health available to us, one that depends more on our nonphysical self. Disease becomes part of our health if it leads us to a life where we are more at peace with ourselves and our relationships and more certain of our goals.[1] Pain can either awaken us into seeing differently or blind us to all but our suffering. Even long-term suffering may end when we finally understand what our inner health is and where to find it.

RESTRUCTURING OUR PARTS

Although our core health is something we have, not a state that we acquire, knowing this does us little good unless we experience this basic truth and claim it as our identity so that we can draw strength from it. Claiming this deeper health requires restructuring our "person parts" so that we have a new and different sense of being whole, one not so dependent on the physical. These include not only our mind, body, and spirit parts but also our roles and goals, our past and future, our fantasies and hopes—all facets of the self, which is "multidimensional."[2] When any of these are seriously threatened or diminished by illness or loss, we experience pain and distress.[3] We suffer.

In a broad sense, what suffering is to many people is getting what they do not want and wanting what they do not get or have. Freud held that "Suffering comes from three quarters: from our own body...from the outer world, which can rage against us with...forces of destruction; and finally, from our relations with other men."[4]

So for Harvard professor and preacher Peter Gomes, the question is: "How do we deal with the fact that inevitably we die, that our life before we die is conflicted and besieged, and that we find it difficult to get along with our fellow creatures? These are not Freudian categories; this is life itself."[5]

DAX COWART'S STORY

Donald "Dax" Cowart, at age 25, was besieged by all three of Freud's suffering forces. He was so severely damaged in just about every part that made him the person he was that he suffered mightily and begged to die. Out of his ordeal, he was left with two plastic eyeballs in sockets where his seeing eyes once were, a skin-grafted "mask" where his face was, and two stumps where his hands and fingers were. Most of the physical parts that once gave him his identity and health are gone. But Dax Cowart, the restructured *person,* is still here.

Survivor of a propane gas explosion in the summer of 1973, Cowart spent 14 long months of painful treatment at three Texas hospitals, including one at my homebase in the Texas Medical Center. From the first horrifying minutes of running through three walls of fire coming out of the massive explosion near Kilgore, Texas, Cowart was in such pain he begged to die. The first request he made of the farmer who heard him screaming on the country road where he lay writhing on the ground was for a gun. "Can't you see I'm a dead man?" Cowart muttered. "I want to put myself out of my misery." The farmer refused and summoned help.

The agonizing, relentless debridements doctors did over the long months ahead to remove foreign material and damaged tissue to save his life were "like being skinned alive." Cowart demanded that treatment stop and that he be allowed to die. When his protests went unheeded, he twice tried to commit suicide but failed from being too weak to kill himself. Literally skin and bones, he weighed 85 pounds. His case has become a textbook classic on medical ethics and the clash between individual rights and social responsibility.

Although his life was saved and he was left with enough of a body that he could walk and talk, Cowart "languished through years of virtual helplessness until he finally began to build a new personal identity," which included a new first name, "Dax."[6] Cowart wanted to die not only because the treatments were so painful but because "I didn't want to live blind and crippled." He had been a high school athlete, a rodeo rider, an Air Force fighter pilot, a man who loved being active outdoors, and one who also enjoyed the party scene. Now he could be or do none of these.

REBUILDING AN IDENTITY

Cowart had to rebuild his person parts, to become whole in a new way, and to find a different kind of health. Money and recognition failed to give him a new identity. He became financially secure from an out-of-court settlement with the energy company whose leaking pipeline caused the accident, which not only maimed Cowart but killed his father who was with him.

Cowart finally managed to graduate from law school, but he never got caught up in a vision of where he was heading until, some years later, he attended a trial lawyers' institute in Wyoming and landed a job with a law firm in Corpus Christi specializing in personal injury.[7] Cowart has also discovered a spiritual side in himself as part of his changed identity and now reads and writes poetry.[8] What continues to give purpose to his life is his advocacy of patients' rights. He speaks before large medical audiences and informs physicians and nurses about patients' legal rights to refuse treatment and to die.

Now, almost 25 years after the explosion, Cowart considers himself "happier than most people I'm around" and has a sense of being well inside himself. Cowart has found a sense of satisfaction and purpose in life, but he still insists that his rights as a patient were ignored and that he should have been allowed to die when he was in such pain.

ACQUIRING EQUANIMITY

A mind at peace with all below . . . .

—BYRON

Physical pain is only one cause of suffering, which can also come from "loss of loved ones, business reversals, prolonged illness, profound injuries to self-esteem, and other damage to personhood."[9] Another man I know, once a student of mine, had his self-esteem severely challenged as a young college freshman, and he too wanted to die until he discovered his inner health. Years before Dr. Dean Ornish became internationally known for demonstrating that life-threatening heart disease can be reversed without drugs or surgery, he had to save his own life.[10] As a freshman at Rice University, a highly competitive, top-ranked school, he was seriously considering suicide because his self-perceived identity as a budding genius had been shattered by the discovery that a number of his peers seemed brighter and excelled with ease while and he had to struggle just to make passing grades in chemistry. Dean's parents had high expectations of him, as is suggested by the name they gave him.

Depressed and physically ill, Ornish went home to his parents in Dallas and was surprised to meet a guest there who was a swami from India, Sri Swami Satchidananda. He was struck by the man's equanimity and quiet strength and understood immediately that this was an inner peace and power he sorely needed. The swami introduced Ornish to meditation, and it changed his life. He discovered an inner health he didn't know he had because it was buried beneath all his frantic striving and fear of not being first. Returning to school the next semester with a source of renewal he could draw on each day, Ornish not only completed his degree at Rice but graduated near the top of his class.

As a student at Baylor College of Medicine, where I met Dean when he did an independent study with me at the UT School of Public Health, he was given permission to teach heart patients stress management techniques and ways to change to a low-fat diet in an attempt to reverse their disease. Ornish went on to become a medical researcher who has done landmark studies showing that people with severe atherosclerosis can reverse their disease using meditation, yoga, group support, exercise, and a very low-fat diet.[11]

FINDING WHAT WE ALREADY HAVE

There is God's laughter on the hills of space
and the happiness of children
and the soft healing of innumerable
dawns and evenings, and the blessing of peace.

—EUGENE O'NEILL

If our inner health is something we already have, not something we have to get, why aren't we more aware of its presence and making use of it? Ornish's answer is that we are too caught up in external distractions that keep us from discovering the peace and joy of subjective well-being. People believe "that their happiness comes from outside themselves," so we keep pursuing false external gods we mistakenly think will give us happiness.[12] Ornish suggests that if we just calmed our mind and body enough to experience "what we have all the time"—an intrinsic health— we'd find the peace and joy we seek.

"An *inner* sense of peace, self-worth, and self-esteem," Ornish found, doesn't come "from getting or from doing but simply from *being*."[13] Without this recognition, "we end up running everywhere else looking for this elusive happiness, in the process disturbing the inner joy and peace we could have if we simply quieted down the mind and body enough to experience that."[14]

What keeps us chasing these false gods and illusory goals when we find from experience they are often empty or unfulfilling once we grasp them? Since the start of Ornish's coronary treatment and research program more than a decade ago, he has maintained that we keep up the pursuit to deaden the pain of loneliness and isolation. Patients in his program have built their lives around over-working, smoking, drinking, overeating, and numbing out on tele-vision because as long as they do, their deep feelings of being alone and apart from others are kept out of awareness. To open their con-gested and constricted arteries, they must open their hearts.[15] The physical change depends on a nonphysical overhaul, which comes from changing their priorities, connecting them with others, and letting them truly experience love, both the receiving and giving of it.

When we connect not only with others but with the center of our being, which links us to God and larger realities, we find both peace and joy. Joy is not the same as happiness. It is rarer and deeper. It is a "fullness of well-being" we encounter when we enter the nonphysical realm of who we are.[16] "Joy is akin to holiness not because of some sense of moral perfection or beauty but because both partake of the sense of the whole, of the complete."[17] We feel it when the broken has been made whole.

ADOPTING A WIDE-ANGLE LENS

When we have a condition that is not going to be cured or a pain that won't go away, basing our identity on the nonphysical enlarges our life so there is room for both the pain and peace. Our illness is part of us but a larger part is the attachments we have to others we love and care about; to service that fulfills us; to music, art, and lit-erature that lift us; to a world of nature that gives us beauty; to a God who strengthens us; and to a universe that is a source of ever-lasting wonder. We adopt a wide-angle lens so we can see there is order and beauty and joy to be experienced as well as pain. We see the pain from a different view, and it looks smaller.[18]

I had a dream one night that let me know I could be "defective," have a "hole" in one part of me and still belong to others and feel at home in the world. I didn't speak plainly as a child and once I became aware of the mispronunciations in my "baby talk," I became self-conscious and lost spontaneity. One day, when I was 6 or 7, a neighborhood adolescent did me the great service, though in a teasing way, of pointing out that I was saying "treek" when I meant "creek." I reddened and went home embarrassed but informed. My mother confessed that she hadn't corrected my mispronunciations because "people think they are cute." In the dream I had I was again misusing sounds and syllables, but people still understood me and didn't laugh at me, and I wasn't shamed by something that in the dream I couldn't change. I awoke with a sense that brokenness and imperfection are part of our "surface" life, which may be turbulent and chaotic, but underneath there is order that binds us to a health large enough to accommodate pain side by side with well-being.

"Is not disease the rule of existence?" Henry David Thoreau asked.[19] Sooner or later, we are all blemished by something on the material or physical level. "There is not a lily pad floating on the river but has been riddled by insects," Thoreau said. "Almost every shrub and tree has its gall, oftentimes esteemed its chief ornament and hardly to be distinguished from the fruit."[20]

In other words, there is still beauty to be seen if we have the eyes for it. "Perfect Leaf" was a game a woman who discovered such eyes played as a small child with her sister. The goal was to go into the backyard and "search diligently for a leaf on any tree or shrub that was perfect. The first person to find one was the winner." The game would go on for hours, particularly in late summer and fall, without a winner. "By then almost all the leaves were imperfect—chewed by insects, shriveled on the edges, marred in endless ways." But what Perfect Leaf taught her was that "beauty and ugliness, perfection and imperfection, can coexist—not only in the same leaf, but probably in ourselves as well."[21]

More to Life Than Pain

To see a World in a Grain of Sand
And a Heaven in a Wild Flower
Hold Infinity in the palm of your hand
And Eternity in an hour.

—BLAKE

Dr. David Spiegel of Stanford conducted a groundbreaking study showing that women with metastatic breast cancer who participate in group therapy and self-hypnosis live twice as long (36 months) as those who get only standard care.[22] He tells of the success that one of his patients, Barbara, had using a wide-angle lens on her life. Her husband had just been diagnosed with Alzheimer's disease. "She was overwhelmed with misery. She had just come to terms with her own cancer...and had been planning a happy period of retirement and freedom to pursue creative activities. She felt imprisoned by her life, unable to escape the endless worries that beset her."[23] Then, under hypnosis, she agreed to look at her concerns from a different point of view, as though "through a camera with a telephoto and a wide-angle lens. She could thus make what she was looking at bigger or smaller, either focusing on it intensely or placing it in a broader context." Barbara began to notice she was not feeling as overwhelmed by her problems. "I realize," she said, "that my illness and my husband's illness are just part of my life—there's more to my life than that."[24]

If we are able to expand our caring center enough so that we see what else we have to absorb us beyond our pain and distress, we will widen our experience of life. To do this, we need the full power of our life force. Western science concluded more than a century ago that the life force is a philosophical abstraction, not a physiological reality. But a number of scientists and clinicians in the West continue to believe "that there is a life force, a spirit or a soul that breathes life into bodies."[25] They see the soul as organizing the life process itself and animating us as persons, each of us unique. Dr. Max Delbruck, a Nobel-Prize–winning molecular biologist and physicist, argued that Aristotle's concept of soul as a life-organizing principle was actually the DNA code, which was discovered 2,500 years later.[26] The soul was just as invisible to Aristotle as the DNA *code* of life is to modern scientists. But both are profoundly real in their effects.

SCIENCE, SOUL, AND PASSION

Whether we are talking about the soul or DNA, we are referring to a core level of our spiritual and physical being. These two realms are not separate, just as religion and philosophy must join at the deepest level. The most advanced theories of science see us joined by universal energy fields (Chapter 2) or, as theoretical biologist Rupert Sheldrake (see Chapter 8) would have it by "morphic fields," in which there is not a transfer of energy but information—an intelligence—that organizes our molecules, cells, tissues, organisms.[27]

When we touch that deepest level of being and existence, whether from a profoundly moving experience, a flash of insight, or intuition, we feel the truth of it in our bones, with a profound effect on all levels. Candace Pert (see Chapter 2) sees the effect, for instance, at the very level of our cells, transmitted there by neuropeptides, small proteins found all over the body and "carriers" of emotion. Unexplainable, spontaneous remissions of metastatic cancer may take place at this deep intersection of soul experience

and cellular effect. Pert's scientific journey has led her from no religion to "a very strong spiritual inclination."[28] In her view, "all the
information in the universe," whether scientific or spiritual, "is
available to all the other information in the universe, and that, to
me, is God."

Is "Soul" Coming Out of the Closet?

The one thing in the world, of value,

is the active soul.

—EMERSON

Despite the endorsement of soul by some scientists, *soul* is not a
word with any standing in the medical and psychological literature. In a secular society that rightly values the accomplishments
of Western science, *soul* is not a word used frequently in conversations of lay people either. But even for the secular, life-threatening
illness may lead to soul recognition. As Anatole Broyard (Chapter
2), who did not consider himself religious, observed after he got
cancer, "I used to get restless when people talked about soul, but
now I know better. Soul is the part of you that you summon up in
emergencies... you don't need to be religious to believe in souls
or to have one."[29]

The soul, spirit, and life force constitute our nonphysical or
"invisible" self. It is essential to a passion for life. Drs. John James
and Muriel James, in their book, *Passion for Life,* hold that "whether
or not we are conscious of the spiritual self, and whether or not we
are open to its power, the spiritual self is the center of our
being... and is part of the natural inheritance with which we are

born."[30] For those who believe that "the existence of the human spirit is a matter of conjecture," that nobody has ever seen it or proved its existence scientifically, the Jameses point out that "like gravity, the spiritual self cannot be seen or touched, but it can be known" and felt.[31] Harvard lecturer Lewis Hyde says we have a spiritual thirst that must be satisfied.[32] It is "the thirst of the self to feel that it is part of something large . . . it is the thirst to grow, to ripen"—in the sense that Alice Trillen (Chapter 3) was using it when she said her life was "very rich," based on the line from King Lear: "Ripeness is all."[33]

MORE THAN MOLECULES IN MOTION

In our proper motion we ascend

Up to our native seat; descent and fall

To us is adverse.

—MILTON

As Aristotle indicated, and the recent work of quantum field physicists is also suggesting, the soul is an intelligence that guides our life force and animating energy. Each individual soul is a nanocosm, "a splinter," as Carl Jung wrote, of a larger, universal intelligence that is the "infinite deity."[34] Christians attach a human face to the infinite intelligence in their 2,000-year-old belief that God became incarnate in the form of Jesus Christ. In the Judaic tradition, there is a Hasidic saying that "all souls are one. Each is a spark of the original soul, and this soul is inherent in all souls."[35]

Our soul and our spirit, our organizing and animating breath of life, enliven us as long as we keep caring and connected. They leave us as we die. If, as many scientists believe, the human organism is nothing but a collection of molecules that are in motion until it dies, then there is no good explanation for why we have a distinct sense that even before the body is dead, the soul and spirit, "the real person," may already be gone. At hospice when I am sitting with a dying person who just the week before was sitting up in bed, eyes bright, talking to friends and family but now is unresponsive, lying with head cocked back, mouth open, breathing heavily, eyes either closed or staring vacantly at the ceiling, it is clear that the life force has largely departed, leaving behind a frail frame that once housed a person with identity and spirit.

Dr. Leon Kass of the University of Chicago, who is both a physician with a Ph.D. in biochemistry and an ethicist, speaks of the soul as "some kind of center of organized power" underlying our personhood and consciousness that may leave by degrees before the rest of us dies.[36] He also reminds us that what "we would call the distinctively human in human life," our personhood and consciousness, is found only "when it's connected with a living, breathing, digesting body."[37] We are, then, embodied spirits, but ones that cannot be accounted for on a strictly physical basis.

WHERE DOES THE "I" IN "I AM" GO?

Some time at eve when the tide is low,

I shall slip my mooring and sail away.

—ELIZABETH CLARK HARDY

What happens to the soul when the body dies? Most scientists would not consider this a proper question, since they would argue there is no empirical evidence proving the soul's existence, much less its destination. But one, Dr. Werner von Braun, was convinced that since "nothing in nature, not even the tiniest particle, can disappear without a trace," the human soul, "the masterpiece" of God's creation, knows no extinction. Like the particle, it too is transformed.[38] It was transformed into the web of oneness that underlies all creation.

But when we see a body cease to breathe and the person who inhabited it "gone," we seldom think about transformation. The question comes back to, "Who am I?" and what happens to the "I" that is "me" when I die? After her own radical mastectomy, chemotherapy, and Tamoxifen (which she is to take for the next five years), Geralyn Wolf of Providence, Rhode Island, a bishop in the Episcopal church, took communion to a parishioner whose breast cancer had recurred. The woman had developed breast cancer at the same age as Wolf, and now, seven years later, the parishioner was dealing with a recurrence.[39]

"So I was hit square in the face with the reality of the power of this disease," says Wolf. . . . I identified with her. I thought, my goodness, what if I died? . . . what would happen to all that I am?" The words *I am* reminded her of what God told Moses in their encounter at the burning bush *(Exodus 3)*. Moses asked, "Who should I say that you are? Who should I say sent me?" God's answer was, "I am who I am." Moses was to tell the Israelites "I am" sent him.

To Wolf, this meant who she is—her "I"—joins the "I am," which is God, when she dies. ". . . this idea was a great comfort, to think of living 'forever in the great I am.' "[40]

NO PHYSICAL EXPLANATION

Strange—is it not?—that of the myriads who
Before us passed the door of Darkness through,
Not one returns to tell us of the road
Which to discover we must travel too.

—OMAR KHAYYAN

Leon Kass tells of going to the hospital room of a man he had visited a number of times, a man whose mind he greatly admired and whose conversation was stimulating and engaging. On the way to the man's room, he asked a nurse, who was coming out, how he was doing. "Didn't you know?" she asked. He died about an hour ago." Kass walked in the room and "there he was...lying in bed, very peaceful....had I not been told by the nurse, I would have taken him as being asleep." Then Kass suddenly found himself on his knees at the end of the bed, "thunderstruck."

> Here he was, but he wasn't there at all.... And all I could think of was—where is he? And where is this mind? What's happened to it?...what was lost was really so great. That, it seems to me, gives anybody pause in thinking that one is going to have an adequate bodily account of what you mean by the human soul.[41]

In instances where death occurs less suddenly, the life force can be so persistent that it may hang on until the last breath while the body dies slowly. The reason for this is that within the life force there is "conatus," a striving power that the 17th Century philosopher Spinoza said that all living creatures are invested with as a means to maintain their existence and state of being. Conatus, like soul, has reached the attention of biological scientists. Molecular biologist Peter Mora wrote a paper in *Nature* in which he said conatus is a persistent "molecular urge."[42] As such, conatus has a material base that may keep a body breathing even after the organizing, animating soul has departed.

John and Elizabeth

This was the case with my friend John Copeland, age 54, who had such resilience he survived a crushed sacrum in 1977 and a massive heart attack nine years later. When a second and fatal myocardial infarction left him without oxygen to the brain for 10 to 12 minutes in 1996, he never regained consciousness but he continued to breathe for more than a week, the last two days without any life support. The person I knew as John looked incredibly the same, even as he lay on his back, eyes closed, struggling for each breath, with his fiancée and friends at his bedside praying and stroking his laboring body.

John was a gifted electrical engineer who used imagery to restore collateral circulation to his oxygen-starved heart after his first heart attack. He was so impressed with the power of the mind to affect the body that he underwent intensive training to become a zen therapist while he did electrical engineering on the side. He was a kind and loving man, who died a few weeks short of his second marriage. The morning he collapsed while moving out of his house to the home he and his new wife would occupy, he managed to make two phone calls: the first to 911 and the second to his future wife, who had gone into a meeting at her office. On her voice mail were his last words: "I called to say I love you."

A year earlier, on August 27, 1995, my wife and I looked at our 31-year-old daughter on her back as she lay on a gurney at the

New York City Medical Examiner's Office. I should say we viewed her body, dead from an overdose of drugs and a fall down 16 hard marble steps in an old hotel, now a seedy apartment house, off upper Amsterdam Avenue. In my wallet was a picture of Liz as I knew her: warm, brown eyes, blonde hair, bright smile, lively expression. Now, without the presence of a soul that organizes and a spirit that animates, her body was there for us to identify, but it was not the person we deeply loved and grieved for. We wept for what was gone, and her death left a long-hurting hole in my midsection, right beneath my heart and surgical hole.

The caring center that connects us with our life force is the guardian of our inner health and the means by which we gain a larger sense of identity and wholeness. When we lose touch with that center, we lose what enlivens us (see Chapter 2). In death the spirit leaves. In depression, it seems to be gone. I have had three major episodes of depression in my life and what has been most terrifying in each is an inability to care. But each time, as I get better, my spirit slowly awakens and my self-identity returns. I have reconnected with my core health. I am myself again. I am well in myself.

Making Sense of Life

Being well in the self is a way of seeing. Such a metaphorical statement has empirical fact to back it up. Being well in oneself involves a sense of coherence, which means we see our life and world as comprehensible, manageable, and meaningful. A strong sense of coherence has been found in repeated studies to be associated with improved quality of life and better biological functioning.[43]

For example, in the study I directed on women who recently completed treatment for breast cancer and participated in a support group or an imagery group, as opposed to only standard care, we found coherence to be an important element in improved life attitudes and a sense of more meaning and purpose. Other research on cancer patients has shown better immune system functioning to be associated with a high sense of coherence.[44]

A sense of coherence, which depends on seeing order in ourselves and our lives, has powerful effects on our central nervous system. It brings the sympathetic branch, which arouses us to fight or flee when faced with life-or-death threats, into balance with the parasympathetic branch, which calms us.

When our sense of coherence is strong, we see our problems as comprehensible. "Death, war, and failure can occur," but we can make sense of them.[45] We also see them as manageable, in the sense that we have resources we can rely on or we know where to turn when we need help to control our problems. "One's spouse, friends, colleagues, God, history... a physician," people we can count on and trust give us guidance, support, and a way to manage.[46]

We also see meaning in the events or our lives, including the bad events. Meaning motivates us and comes out of an active caring center. Without it, a strong sense of coherence is impossible.[47]

A LONG LOOK AND WIDER VIEW

What is essential is invisible to the eye.

—SAINT-EXUPÉRY

The words *see* and *look* punctuate the accounts that cancer patients, permanently injured persons, and others with chronic disorders and disabilities give of their efforts in recovering a healthy identity.[48] They "see" what is important in life. They "look" at themselves differently. They see value in what they used to ignore or take for granted.

As one cancer patient said: "You take a long look at your life and realize that many things you thought were important before are totally insignificant.... You put things into perspective."[49] Lilly, the stage IV cancer patient I mentioned in the previous chapter, said in the interview I had with her that "my view of life was very narrow before I got this illness. Cancer has opened up a new world. You are, I am, really living every day, and we need to stay mindful of the gift we have."[50] Dan Wakefield, a writer who sees living each day as a creative act, asks:

> Do you "go on automatic," move in a kind of waking coma through the rituals of the day? I know how easy it is to fall into these routinized bad habits because I do it myself, unless I pay attention, bring myself back to wakefulness. Most of us dismiss as boring the nitty-gritty of waking, eating, washing the dishes, carrying on relationships with loved ones, paying the bills, answering the phone, solving problems, mowing the grass, tending the garden, feeding the cat, walking the dog, going to bed and to sleep again, waking anew each morning.... Seeing these ordinary activities as part of our creative lives, related to everything else we do, and seeing all we do as *creation* infuses us with power.[51]

A number of women in our study talked about a new perspective in terms of reordering their priorities. One said: "You've heard about no one wanting on their tombstone, 'I wish I had spent more time at the office.' I believe that now. My friends and family are more important to me." Another commented, "I don't want to waste today because tomorrow I may be unable to get out of bed."

A successful investor and environmental activist named W. Mitchell, was disfigured from severe burns suffered in a motorcycle accident in 1971, which left him without fingers and also nearly killed him. Four years later he was in a small plane that crashed, and he was paralyzed from the waist down. He tells people who are dealing with tragedies to step back from their misfortunes and "take a wider view." When he suffered his double dose of injury and pain, he said: "I could choose to see this situation as a setback or a starting point."[52] He chose to see it as a new beginning.

What's Really Important

Dr. Rachel Naomi Remen, medical director of Commonweal Cancer Help Program in California, had a patient, a highly successful businessman, who said that "before his cancer he would become depressed unless things went a certain way." He believed that happiness depended on "having the cookie." Here's how he saw it:

> If you had the cookie, things were good. If you didn't have the cookie, life wasn't worth a damn. Unfortunately, the cookie kept changing. Some of the time it was money, sometimes power, sometimes sex, new car, biggest contract, most prestigious address.... When I give my son a cookie, he is happy. If I take the cookie away or it breaks, he is unhappy. But he is two and a half and I am forty-three. It's taken me this long to understand that the cookie will never make me happy for long. The minute you have the cookie it starts to crumble or you start to worry about it crumbling or about someone trying to take it away from you.[53]

Cancer changed all that. Now he is happy for the first time whether his business is going well or not, whether he wins or loses at golf. He decided that what is really important to him is simply life. "Life any way you can have it."[54] Now he sees that life *is* the cookie. He continues to be free of cancer, Remen told me.[55]

INNER AND OUTER EYES

To rich and poor alike, with lavish hand;

Though most hearts never understand

To take it at God's value, but pass by

The offered wealth with unrewarded eye.

—JAMES RUSSELL LOWELL

Seeing, then, is an attitude as much as sensory sight. It requires both inner and outer eyes. Galileo, whose discoveries in astronomy reflected both, called them, the eye of the mind and the eye of the forehead. Jacques Lusseyran, who became a widely recognized writer and professor, learned to see after he became blind at age 7. He said he learned that seeing is "contemplating" the fact that neither joy nor light comes from without, but from within, and life is a gift given to us by the minute.[56] Lusseyran learned to love what exists, and what existed for him was an inner light.

The Vedas, sacred hymns written in archaic Sanskrit, present to Hindus a world of "blinding splendor" and teach the supreme importance of truly seeing. *Darsan,* the Hindu word for seeing, is what sanctifies the worshiper, who learns that the eye, both inner and outer, is truth.[57] Seeing is a way of communicating with the world, a way of touching and being touched by the light in the darkness.

Wordsworth, Blake, and a host of nature poets have long spoken of our being connected to a grander reality. With the advent of quantum theory, some scientists are speaking the same way. At a meeting of the American Association for the Advancement of

Science, in a remarkable session on "Seeing Ourselves in the Stars," the "hard" scientists present were urged by an astronomer to start paying more attention to poetic insights, because quantum superstring physics posits that there *is* a world in a grain of sand, as Blake insisted, and that there is an intelligent field of energy and order at the most fundamental levels of reality, which includes us and all of nature. Newton, as well as Einstein, was convinced of the existence of a transcendent knowledge beyond humankind that organizes the universe, although we but dimly perceive it.

How We Are Joined

No man is an Iland intire, of it selfe;

every man is a peece of the Continent,

a part of the maine . . . .

—DONNE

When we develop, then, an orientation, an attitude, of seeing, we see that we are all joined, that everything is related to something bigger, and that we live in a "participatory universe," as physicist John Wheeler calls it.[58] But how are we joined? We are joined not only by a fundamental energy and order but by our shared mortality, and "together we construct the rituals, seek the cures, find the means of solace, and fight the indignities of sickness and death," no matter who we are or where.[59] We also see that there are gifts to be found even in darkness. As Marilyn McEntyre has put it: "There is a gift in the dark mine of pain and fear for those who will carry in their picks and find it."[60] For this kind of seeing, we need both the eye of the forehead and the eye of the mind. Author Annie Dillard is among those who use both. She writes:

There are lots of things to see, unwrapped gifts and free surprises. The world is fairly studded and strewn with pennies cast broadside from a generous hand. But . . . who gets excited by a mere penny? If you . . . crouch motionless on a bank to watch a tremulous ripple thrill on the water and are rewarded by the sight of a muskrat kid paddling from its den, will you count that sight a chip of copper only, and go your rueful way? It is dire poverty indeed when a man is so malnourished and fatigued that he won't stoop to pick up a penny. But if you can cultivate healthy poverty and simplicity, so that finding a penny will literally make your day, then, since the world is in fact planted in pennies, you have with your poverty bought a lifetime of days. It is that simple. What you see is what you get.[61]

Those in the remission society and pain fellowship who are well though wounded have the ability to see gifts in many places, even in their own chronic condition and pain. This ability depends on keeping our caring center healthy. By caring beyond our pain we connect to the gifts around us, and in doing so we mobilize not only our life force and spirit but our capacity to heal.

BEING HEALED BUT NOT CURED

Healing is not curing; it is something larger. People in this book have told me that they feel healed but not cured—that is, as a report to the National Institutes of Health puts it, such persons "experience a profound sense of psychological or spiritual well-being and wholeness although the actual disease remains."[62]

Unlike curing, which usually depends on external intervention, "healing is an inner process through which the human organism seeks its own recovery—physically, mentally, emotionally, and spiritually."[63] Healing is what we experience when we succeed in joining together that which is divided in us and our relationships. Just as healing can occur while pain remains, it can take place in the act of dying, as I said earlier. (See also Chapter 10).

One of the ways we help healing to occur is by telling our stories—stories of who we are, what impassions us, what keeps us going when the going gets tough. Stories are not just recitations of the events and activities in our life, many of which are common to everyone, but translations of how we experience what happens to us in life. What starts as inarticulate and inchoate gradually becomes coherent as we talk about, or write, our deepest feelings and thoughts—our experience of life—and begin to perceive the meaning in who we are and why we are here. (See Pennebaker's research in Chapter 9).

Stories connect us not only to other people but to our core self, our center of felt experience and consciousness. If we suffer from an illness and tell our stories to others with that illness, we experience a special connection and freedom from loneliness. Remen discovered this from having Crohn's disease, a chronic, progressive intestinal disorder, from the time she was 15. As a physician she came to discover that the stories of her patients were "more compelling to me than the disease process."[64] They were the way doctor and patient connected at a healing level.

> ...I became deeply moved by these stories, by the people and the meaning they found in their problems, by the unsuspected strengths, the depths of love and devotion.... They would make me proud to be a human being.[65]

Remen reminds us that families used to sit around the kitchen table and tell their stories. It was a way wisdom got passed on, "the stuff that helps us to live a life worth remembering."[66] I myself grew up when families, friends, and neighbors would gather on each other's front porches and swap stories of their lives. I remember my maternal grandfather's stories on playing in circus bands and what it had meant to him. What it meant to me, since he passed on his old baritone horn to me and my brother, was an early start in appreciating how music is a path to a deeper part of the self. I got a glimpse of the healing power of both stories and music.

SITTING WITH LIZ AND HEALING

Rita and I had a chance to heal our relationship with our daughter Liz before she died. We sat at her bedside in the Intensive Cardiac Care Unit of St. Luke's Hospital in New York City and, through tears, laughter, hugs, stories, music, and exchanges of deep sorrow and regrets, we reconnected. We recaptured memories of all the places we had travelled together and the beauty we had seen in the world with her.

We looked at her watercolors, read poetry, listened to Mozart, and let go of years of frustration, anger, crushed hopes, agonizing despair, and sadness. We were told that if she managed to pull through, she would live for maybe two or three years more if she stopped doing drugs. She didn't stop, and she lived for three years.

What good is this kind of healing if death is the outcome anyway? For Liz, she died knowing how deeply she was loved. For Rita, she could accept what was inevitable with some sense of completion. For me, it kept my caring center alive. I escaped depression. I had lost any sense of caring in a deep depression I slowly recovered from two years before we sat with her in the ICU. I thought her impending death would trigger a recurrence. But something changed for me after that experience at her bedside. I still had the deep aching that had been in my belly for years but now I felt a different kind of health, and it has sustained me.

From the cancer patients I have worked with in my research and those I have sat with at hospice, I have been struck by four common denominators to their inner health: appreciation, creative use of pain, faith, and resilience. These are not just my findings, and they do not apply only to persons with cancer. They are common to the healing experienced by many chronically ill persons who see themselves as healthy. The power of these four is beginning to penetrate the consciousness of Western medical science. We will explore each in the chapters that follow and see how they add to both the quality and quantity of our lives.

Chapter Five

APPRECIATING

WHAT IS

I asked for all things that I might enjoy life,
and I was given life, that I might enjoy all things.
I got nothing that I asked for —
but everything I had hoped for.
I am . . . most richly blessed.

—AN UNKNOWN SOLDIER,

CIVIL WAR

M any in the fellowship of pain have discovered that they can have a different kind of health while living with serious illness or disability by appreciating what they have rather than bemoaning what they have lost or will never get. When I asked the women treated for cancer the question "Have you found any value in the experience you have had with your illness?" the most frequent answer boiled down to: "I appreciate life more now." More than a few said they now literally stop to smell the roses, which they seldom noticed before cancer came into their lives.

How Good It Feels

Serious illness teaches most all of us to appreciate. When we recover from being sick, we delight in just functioning again, we feel alive, we marvel at the pleasures of ordinary acts of daily living. To walk across the room or down the hall under our own steam seems wonderful. To stand and look straight across at people as we talk with them, instead of up at them from a sick bed, is so gratifying. We find that "just being alive, on a no-frills basis, is astonishingly good."[1] People write books about how good it feels.[2] We learn to savor life, ordinary life. We have looked into the abyss and we came out believing in life more than ever.

But caught up again in daily living, many of us forget to keep appreciating. We become distracted, we take for granted what seemed so good when we first recovered—or when we were still looking out our hospital window wishing we could just join the busy people on the street going about their activities of living. We stop noticing the roses and go on automatic.

PAYING ATTENTION TO THE ORDINARY

When Dr. Jon Kabat-Zinn introduces stress management to chronic pain patients in his clinic at the University of Massachusetts Medical Center, he often starts by passing around a bowl of raisins and asking each person to pick one, truly look at it, smell it, and chew it slowly, using all the senses to savor it.[3] His point is that we miss so much we could appreciate by eating without truly tasting, by not being mindful and neglecting the ordinary.[4] When he teaches the patients to meditate, they are ready to pay attention to simply following their breath in and out. The program does not "cure" pain or the injury or illness underlying it, but it does offer a way to relieve pain by learning "full catastrophe living." Kabat-Zinn's book by that title is taken from the novel *Zorba the Greek,* who takes catastrophe as part of life and dances in response.

> Zorba's response embodies a supreme appreciation for the richness of life and the inevitability of all its dilemmas, sorrow, tragedies, and ironies. His way is to "dance" in the gale of the full catastrophe, to celebrate life, to laugh with it and at himself, even in the face of personal failure and defeat.[5]

For those of us who don't go on automatic after recovery or remission, who keep mindful of how precious life is from living with the threat that our cancer or other recurring disease will flare up again, appreciation becomes a way of life. It is a way that keeps us in touch with that part of us beyond the ravages of disease.

AWAKENING TO ASTONISHMENT

From the beginning I felt a kinship with nature's offspring—animals, plants, rocks, forests, water, earth, the sky, and even with remote stars and galaxies. No one taught me this; I simply awoke with the conviction of my relatedness to these things.

—RENÉE WEBER

When we feel a deep kinship and connection with the universe we live in, we are responding not only with appreciation but with astonishment. Nobelist Ilya Prigogine, an octogenarian chemist and physicist who is affiliated with both the University of Texas at Austin, which has a center in his name, and a similar research center in Brussels, sees "astonishment" as "what is common to our time."[6] Whether we believe in God or not, Prigogine says, the universe is astonishing.

"Not so long ago," he notes, "people were thinking that with Newton's laws, extended by quantum mechanics and relativity, we knew the universe. Now we see that we know very little." It is so astonishing that within Prigogine's theories of "dissipative structures" he believes that "the beginning of the universe was not the beginning of time, but simply transformation from a pre-universe to a universe," from virtual particles, for instance, to real particles.[7] We don't have to appreciate astonishment, but there is enough beauty that comes with it that gratitude seems to come easy to those who feel a kinship.

Norman Cousins, longtime *Saturday Review* editor who became a lecturer at UCLA Medical School on mind/body medicine, extended both the quantity and quality of his own life through the healing effects of gratitude. He wrote a few years before his death: "An appreciation of life can be a prime tonic for mind and body. Being able to respond to the majesty of the way nature fashions its art" can bring "wondrous satisfactions" as well as healing benefits.[8]

CALMING EFFECTS OF GRATITUDE

Gratitude is the heart's memory.

—FRENCH PROVERB

Recent studies show the power that appreciation has on producing positive effects on both the body and emotions.

Researchers have found that when we get angry or think angry thoughts, the sympathetic branch of the autonomic nervous system (ANS) is activated and causes the heart rate to increase and arteries to constrict, a pattern that is linked to cardiac disease and death.[9]

In contrast, when we think about someone or something we really appreciate and experience that feeling, the parasympathetic—calming—branch of the ANS is triggered. This pattern is believed to bestow a protective effect on the heart. The electromagnetic heart patterns of volunteers tested become more coherent, more ordered, when they activate feelings of appreciation.

What this means is that in the midst of stress or anger, pausing to focus on something we deeply appreciate restores balance in the autonomic nervous system and reduces blood pressure.[10] Pausing to appreciate is called the "Freeze-Frame" technique. People are asked to recognize stressful or angry moments, then—as if they are pushing the pause button on a movie camera—stop and shift attention to their hearts and something they are grateful for.

There is evidence, based on controlled studies by a research group in Boulder Creek, California, that when we practice a technique of bringing to attention what we appreciate in our life, more positive emotions emerge, leading to beneficial "alterations in heart rate variability," which may not only relieve hypertension but reduce the risk of sudden death from coronary artery disease.[11] The more we pause to appreciate and show caring and compassion, the more order and coherence we experience internally, which leads to a healthy heart rate variability. A flexible, but ordered, heart rate variability is important because as we face changing conditions, such as stress and exertion, we need the heart rate to vary in response to the demands we are facing. We also want it to return promptly to baseline when the demands cease. When we and our hearts are in an "internal coherence state," studies suggest, we enjoy the capacity to be peaceful and calm yet retain the ability to respond appropriately to stressful circumstances.[12] The concept of being internally coherent as proposed by the California researchers is consistent with Antonovsky's measures of a personal "sense of coherence" (Chapters 3 and 4) that is defined by the degree to which we make sense of life and see it as meaningful and manageable. As we noted, a strong sense of coherence is associated with an improved quality of life and improved biological functioning, including immune competence.

Gratitude may be good for us for other reasons as well. Dr. Timothy Miller, whose book, *How to Want What You Have,* instructs us on the value of gratitude and says that when we stop to appreciate, we often have the urge to say "thank you." When we gratefully thank someone, we often smile. Research I cited in *Who Gets Sick* shows that smiling may reset the autonomic nervous system so that it is less reactive to stress.[13] One study shows that a facial expression of happiness, which is often prompted by gratitude, can increase blood flow to the brain and stimulate release of beneficial neurotransmitters.[14]

Gratitude is also good for us, I believe, because it helps fulfill our basic yearning to feel part of something larger than the self. Out of the 3 million visitors to Westminster Abbey every year, the most openly expressed appreciation comes from those who attend Evensong services. They experience being touched at soul level by the extraordinary fusion of sound and light. The 22 superb voices of the Boys Choir blend beautifully with the beams of fading afternoon light streaming through the ancient abbey windows. The Very Reverend Michael Mayne, who retired as Dean after 10 years at Westminster, said that this experience of transcendence was not only his most abiding memory of his time there but it was also what visitors told him they most appreciated hearing and seeing.[15]

Some rare human beings are able to derive such gratitude for life itself that even when that life is very brief, they feel deep appreciation. The most grateful patient Dr. Alan Blum, a colleague at the Texas Medical Center, has had is a woman who gave birth to a baby born with anencephaly, a condition in which head and brain is so small that it is hardly more than a knob at the top of the spinal cord.

Tests showed while she was pregnant that she was carrying a baby with such a disorder, and she was told he would not likely live long. She wanted the baby to be born anyway. Twelve minutes after birth, the tiny boy died. "He lived long enough to be born, to be held by his grandparents, to be held by me, and to die in my arms," the mother said. She had nothing but appreciation for those who helped her fulfill these hopes and only gratitude for her baby's brief life itself.[16]

"Real World" Benefits

The California researchers who test the effects of appreciation work with very materialistic corporate types who are bottom-line oriented and are not accustomed to pausing and thinking of something they are grateful for. But because such a method produces results for the heart both emotionally and physically, it holds promise of reducing stress and keeping tense people calmer and better able to think straight and make good decisions in the business world. Learning both to appreciate and to meditate produces practical outcomes in the everyday world of making a living as well as making a life worth living.

Just as Ornish found that meditation helped him succeed materially as well as spiritually and emotionally, a few corporate entrepreneurs and chief executive officers have also made meditating a part of their daily discipline. They are different from most of their fellow CEOs, who—like my many colleagues in academia and friends in business—look at meditation as a retreat inward that is likely to be irrelevant, if not antithetical, to the "real world" of competition and "getting ahead."

Jirka Rysavy is the founder and CEO of Corporate Express, a $3.2 billion office-supply Fortune 500 company based outside of Boulder, Colorado, which employs 23,000 people worldwide. He started meditating in 1982 in his native Czechoslovakia and discovered meditation gave him a creativity and self-confidence that enabled him to start from the bottom in this country in 1984 and climb rapidly to the top.

Meditation, he says, is central to his life.[17] He considers it as providing his "internal disciplines" as well as an experience of "unity."[18] His company's new 160,000-square-foot world head-quarters reflects Rysavy's emphasis on unity with the environment. "Once you experience the unity with other things, you come naturally to protect the environment," he says. His company is located at 1 Environmental Way in Broomfield, Colorado, and stresses environmentally safe products, which carry an "Earthsaver" logo.

Rysavy's "unity with other things" is experienced not only in his daily meditation practice but in the way he lives. He has a small house on 110 acres in the mountains above Boulder, which he bought in 1985, and where he loves watching the mountain lions, bears, and deer roam. His meditation enhances his inner health. Daily runs are for his outer health.

BLESSED AND BELOVED

So are you to my thoughts as
Food to Life
Or as sweet-season'd showers
Are to the ground.

—SHAKESPEARE

We have seen that inner health comes from perceiving in ourselves and the world a coherence and order that are deeper than the chaos and disorder that are more visible and measurable in both ourselves and the life around us. The coherence and order we discern depend on identifying with a wholeness larger than the body, a life of maintaining healthy personal relationships, of staying in communion with nature and God, of keeping stimulated in mind and spirit, of feeling at home in the universe.

My life with Rita is what has drawn me to wholeness. Because I was able to first taste wholeness through her, I have been able to survive severe depressions and gradually nourish that core part of me with a growing passion for life. Poet Raymond Carver, who gave up a wild life of hard drinking and hard living for his beloved Tess, married her after they had been together for 11 years and he was diagnosed with lung cancer from a heavy smoking habit that finally caught up with him. He was 50 at the time.

In his last poems, Carver expressed an appreciation that captures what we feel when we say we are "blessed." In the year before he died, he and Tess Gallagher were sitting on their deck one day, taking stock of their lives while looking out on the Strait of Juan de Fuca off the Washington Coast. This is how Tess recalls their conversation in that final year when Carver's cancer went to the brain and recurred in the lungs:

> "You remember telling me how you almost died before you met me?" I asked him. "It could've ended back then and we'd never even have met. None of this would have happened." We sat there quietly, just marveling at what we'd been allowed. "It's all been gravy," Ray said. "Pure gravy."[19]

"Gravy" became the title of one of the fine, short poems that Carver wrote as he neared life's end. It begins:

> No other word will do. For that's what it was. Gravy.
> Gravy, these past ten years.
> Alive, sober, working, loving and
> being loved by a good woman . . . .

And it ends with:

. . . I'm a lucky man.
I've had ten years longer than I or anyone
expected. Pure gravy. And don't forget it.[20]

Carver's appreciation of life couldn't be separated from his
deep love for Tess, as I can't separate mine from my love for Rita.
He looks out the window and sees her bending to cut roses from
the bushes "given for our late wedding" and named, Love, Honor,
and Cherish. She brings him a rose from Cherish.

. . . I press
my nose to it, draw the sweetness in, let it cling—scent
of promise, of treasure. My hand on her wrist to bring her close, her
eyes green as river-moss. Saying it then, against
what comes: *wife,* while I can, while my breath, each hurried petal
can still find her.[21]

Carver's writing, Gallagher noted, "had enabled him to reach
far beyond the often mean circumstances from which he and those
he wrote about had come, out of working-class lives.[22] Gallagher
said that "on a piece of paper near his typewriter he had written:
'Forgive me if I'm thrilled with the idea, but just now I thought
that every poem I write ought to be called Happiness.'" Carver
never expected to feel himself "beloved," but that was his final accomplishment, which he acknowledged in his last poem:

And did you get what
you wanted from this life, even so?
I did.
And what did you want?
To call myself beloved, to feel myself
beloved on this earth.[23]

MINING GOOD FROM THE BAD?

If we appraise our life as a whole, we will see that there is more to it than our chronic illness or pain. We will find many gifts to appreciate even in the midst of great hardship. One compelling piece of evidence that supports such a thesis comes from a study of concentration camp prisoners. Those who survived and stayed healthiest after liberation developed a coping style called "the differential focus on the good."[24] Disease, death, and brutality were all around them. But to stay sane and strong internally, they found "good" to focus on: the beauty of sunrises and sunsets, the bonding with sympathetic listeners, the exchange of memories and stories, the discovery of an unclaimed potato in the field, the blessing of getting through the food line without being beaten, the conviction that they had loved ones to live for, the belief that their God would give them strength to survive.

Dirk Stronck, now a Houston businessman, spent three years of his childhood in labor camps after the Japanese moved in on Malaya and Thailand and took Singapore. He and his Dutch mother and father, together with his brother, were imprisoned. His father was sent to a separate camp, where he died. Stronck remembers that the women in his camp, including his mother, formed a chorus and orchestra, which kept up their spirits.[25] Stronck was able to raise a small garden, and he learned to appreciate the gifts of natural beauty. His mother, who died three years ago, taught him in the camp to find some good in the bad. He remembers what she had taught her small son to focus on.

> It didn't matter if there was one flower, she would say, "Look how beautiful the flowers are. Look how beautiful the stars are. Look how the moon is on the river." It's with me 24 hours a day.[26]

At age 67, Stronck says he is still "in awe of the sunrise and the trees and leaves."[27]

Appreciating what we have that is good when we are struggling hard against what is bad requires suspending the judgments in our head that insist it's crazy to look for a ray of light in stormy skies that are dumping havoc into our lives. The same critical inner voice also tells us, outside of the storms and crises, that there is nothing special about smelling a rose and appreciation is not to be wasted on the ordinary. My acquaintance with illness and pain has taught me to delight in the ordinary: walking the dog, reading the newspaper, sipping coffee, watching sunsets, waiting for the dawn.

HARMONY IN THE MIDST OF NOISE

One meaning of appreciation is "perceptions of delicate impressions or distinctions."[28] If we look closely enough at the ordinary, we often find something distinctive to appreciate. Something bigger is often manifested in something smaller and mundane. We can experience a "sense sublime" in watching the sky brighten at dawn, as Wordsworth did.[29] Appreciation is "a kind of knowing that is different from the mind's way of categorizing, classifying and judging," psychologist Donald Klein reminds us.[30] It is, again, a way of seeing.

A differential focus on the good is an appreciation of the background of harmony that we can find even in the presence of a foreground of noise. Paying attention to what is good in my life does not mean I ignore my pain. It means that when I keep mindful of the connections I have with a larger wholeness and order, I can often lift myself out of my pain or relieve it. My communion with nature is something I feel deeply, right down to the bone. I believe strongly in the "biophilia hypothesis," which holds that humans have "a deep, genetically based emotional need to affiliate with the rest of the living world. Meeting this need ... may be as important to human well-being as forming close personal relationships."[31]

MOUNTAINS AND BIOPHILIA

Full many a glorious morn have I seen
Flatter the mountain-tops with sovereign eye,
Kissing with golden face the meadows green,
Gilding pale streams with heavenly alchemy.

—SHAKESPEARE

I "affiliate" best in the mountains. I take great delight in watching for the first wildflowers of spring, particularly in the Colorado Rockies, where Rita and I have hiked, backpacked, and climbed for years. I love to watch for the first dandelions, the "lowlies" of the floral kingdom. They break through the snow early, liberating winter's hold and heralding the high color to come. In the bright spring sun they soon spread a yellow carpet across mountainsides and valleys.

The lowlies help sustain me because they give me appreciation of a life-death-life cycle that characterizes all that exists. After dandelions have their day in the sun, beautifying the slopes and meadows, they become gossamer "puff balls," blown by the mountain winds to far-off places, where they start life over again. I appreciate and take comfort in the natural law that tells me that new life springs from death, that when I have to give up people and things I love (or habits I cling to), I will feel pain but I will make room for new growth in my life and can look forward to some greening and sprouting ahead. When I die physically, my hope is that I will leave something of myself behind from which new energy and life will be generated. I have found that if I stay mindful of the little things, the lowlies around me, I will better appreciate that all of us are lowlies in a grander order to which we and all life belong.

AN OLD FRIEND ON A RAINY DAY

Dear common flower, that grow'st beside the way,
Fringing the dusty road with harmless gold!
—JAMES RUSSELL LOWELL

Plants often give me unexpected pleasure when I need most to lighten up. I remember a day in the rain after we had left our daughter Liz in ICU at St. Luke's Hospital in New York and walked under our umbrellas in the gardens outside the massive Gothic Cathedral of St. John the Divine, a block down Amsterdam Avenue. On the church grounds is a biblical garden where plants named in the scriptures grow inside an old fence with an iron gate. I was pleased to find among the neatly tagged botanical specimens *Taraxacum officinale,* my old friend the dandelions. The fact that they are in an early book *(Exodus)* of the Hebrew Bible gave me a sense of connecting to something good and grounded that endures.

A story is told of an urban dweller who had used all kinds of lawn treatments to eliminate dandelions from her beautiful front yard grass. Finally, she wrote an expert at the Department of Agriculture, saying she had tried everything and wondered if there was anything else she could do. The reply: "Yes, try learning to love them."

Dorothy and Bobbie

The world is too much with us; late and soon,

Getting and spending, we lay waste our powers:

Little we see in Nature that is ours;

We have given our hearts away, a sordid boon!

—WORDSWORTH

Cancer patients I have met, interviewed, and done research on often mention appreciating the mundane offerings of life they used to ignore. From their illness they have learned to change the way the world looks to them by accepting with gratitude the pleasures of ordinary existence.

Dorothy, 53, came down with Crohn's disease (see Remen in Chapter 4) shortly after she underwent a modified radical mastectomy for cancer and had excruciating bowel pain. Now with some relief from that pain, she is learning to "enjoy every minute to the fullest," and, she told me, "I am getting better at it."[32] Before her cancer and Crohn's disease, she felt guilty if she weren't *doing* something every minute, keeping busy, working hard. Now she lets herself enjoy *being*—being with her flowers, with her friends and family, with her cats. She sees appreciation as a "need." And what she needed was to learn to slow down—which both her illnesses have taught her to do—so she could appreciate what she has in life.

Bobbie Thorne, a white-haired cancer survivor I met at a seminar on cancer remissions, learned to "wake up each morning with thanks and joy" instead of dread of another day. "I wake up remembering 'this is the day the Lord has made, be glad in it.' "[33] Eighteen months earlier she had gone to Commonweal, which offers educational and support programs for persons with cancer and other serious illnesses. She learned yoga and meditation but most of all she acquired a "new vision" of the way the world is. "Even if I don't survive my cancer, I feel healed. I found a oneness, a unity, a wholeness, I didn't know before." To Ms. Thorne, and many like her, these words are not vague abstractions, without concrete meaning. She found that compassion, gratitude, and beauty join us together in experiencing a unity. She learned that there is a larger reality to interact with, which is the source of unity and wholeness. When Ms. Thorne started having severe abdominal pain, she thought, "Is this it, the beginning of the end?" However tests showed no recurrence, only adhesions from her cancer surgery. After Commonweal, Ms. Thorne began working with cancer support groups in Pennsylvania to offer what she had learned from her own experience.

Psychologist Klein says he finds unity in appreciation, which he experiences as "the total feeling of oneness with the universe that I recall having as a child when I kicked my way through rustling piles of autumn leaves. It is the sheer joy of being alive in the world."[34]

MEDITATION AND THE INNER WORLD

There is no man alone, because every man is a microcosm, and carries the whole world about him.

—SIR THOMAS BROWNE

The feeling of being connected to a larger whole has been the experience reported by many who learn to meditate. As Frederic Buechner puts it in *Listening to Your Life:*

> We do our twenty minutes of meditation a day in the hope that, properly stilled, our minds will stop just reflecting back to us the confusion and multiplicity of our world but will turn to a silvery mist like Alice's looking glass that we can step through into a world where the beauty that sleeps in us will come awake at last.[35]

Meditation, as Dr. James Gordon of Georgetown Medical School sees it, is "not simply about quieting the autonomic nervous system and decreasing pain. It is basically a way of being with oneself and the world. It brings a new perspective."[36] Practicing mindfulness meditation, a technique that focuses on following one's breath in and out, taught me to live with more awareness of the pleasures that mundane moments of life can bring.

In the mindfulness method, the most basic, ordinary function of the body—breathing—is used to teach us to look at what we take for granted. What we find when we learn to look—whether at a flower, a tree, a bite of food, a baby, or our breath—is joy and gratitude that at some deep core of all that exists, we are not isolated and separate but members of one another. Plato said that paying attention, truly looking and listening, is a form of love, and perhaps that is one reason meditation connects us to our inner health.

People who have suffered life-threatening illnesses report that having someone to love and be loved by stands near the top of what they appreciate.[37] Many say they took for granted their spouses, families, and friends and are now once again paying attention, truly looking and listening in relating to others so that love is being valued. In the Recurrent Coronary Prevention Project at Mount Sinai Hospital in San Francisco, participants who reorder their values and "plant spiritual gardens"—giving priority to love, beauty, the gift of life itself—significantly reduce their risk of premature death from recurring heart attacks.[38]

JAMES LEE BYARS' THANKS

Instead of complaining that God has hidden himself, you should give him thanks for having revealed so much of himself.

—PASCAL

Expressing gratitude for life itself can have surprising healing effects and restore us to the land of the living. Such was the experience of James Lee Byars, an internationally known sculptor and performance artist whose work has been exhibited at the Museum of Modern Art and the Guggenheim in New York. He was diagnosed with abdominal cancer in 1990 and underwent surgery at Memorial Sloan-Kettering Hospital.[39] Told that he had only a few years to live, Byars moved back to his hometown of Santa Fe to live out his final years. A second operation was then necessary, which led to his being placed on a respirator and undergoing intensive drug therapy. A month later he was transferred to a nursing home, where he expected to die. A nurse suggested to Byars that he might want to visit with Dr. Tony Rippo, a physician who cofounded the Santa Fe Institute for Medicine and Prayer. When Rippo went to the nursing home, Byars struck the physician as "a typical nursing home patient who sits in a wheelchair all day."[40]

Byars said to him, "I'm afraid to die. Can you help me?" Rippo asked him to talk about his fears. Then he gave Byars a mantra: "Lord, thank you for my life." Byars said, "I didn't believe it at first, but it was simple and positive—so I said it. I found that repeating it reduced my fears." A short time later, Byars stopped all his pain medication, became more alert, and in three months he went home. "Now, I really do feel grateful for my life, and I want to work again."[41] Byars did just that and died on May 23, 1997, in Cairo, Egypt at age 65.

CLOSE BRUSHES WITH DEATH

. . . flying waters descending straight . . .

—LI PO

I often use a mantra of gratitude in my daily prayers. What I repeat is, "I praise God for the blessings of this life" and "I thank the Lord for his grace." Gratitude for life gushes out of us when we have sudden, close brushes with death. I have come close to losing my life twice in the mountains. On a summer climb above Blue Lake in the Indian Peaks Wilderness, I lost my footing transversing a large snow field covering the mountainside. I was sliding helplessly down the steep slope when my boots suddenly hit a rock and stopped me. Slowly, I managed to work my way back up to where Rita, with firmer footing, was holding out a saving hand to help pull me to her.

The second time was three years later, on the day before my birthday, when I foolishly tried to use a largely collapsed wooden bridge to cross the roaring Middle Boulder Creek, surging down the mountain with record runoff from heavy winter and spring snows. My foot slipped on the steeply angled wet boards, and I fell within 12 inches of the dangling bridge's edge, overlooking a 10-foot drop to the raging water crashing on the boulders below. What saved me was a large knothole in one of the boards that had made up the floor of the bridge. I hit on my left shoulder and managed to grab the knothole with my right hand. I was then able to throw one leg over the top of the board I was clinging to and scramble to safety. The gratitude I immediately felt for being alive was overwhelming. The appreciation that came afterward was, first, for just being alive, and second, for the fragility of my life, realizing the suddenness with which it can end.

———◆———

BEAUTY AS A PHYSICAL FORCE

A day so happy.

Fog lifted early, I worked in the garden.

Hummingbirds were stopping

over honeysuckle flowers.

There was no thing on earth

I wanted to possess . . . .

To think that once I was the same man

did not embarrass me.

In my body I felt no pain . . . .

—CZESLAW MILOSZ

Keeping in awareness how tenuous life is helps me to remember the ancient advice to live each day as if it is your last. Bringing some beauty into every day of my life helps me to follow this maxim. I want each day, including my last, to have beauty in it, for with beauty I experience my inner health most strongly and appreciate life more. Beauty is a physical force. We catch our breath in its presence. It moves us viscerally. The very word *aesthetics* is derived from the term for "I gasp."[42] The physician-psychologist Havelock Ellis was convinced that "when we are talking aesthetics, we are ultimately talking physiologically."[43] Beauty has a wholeness, a unity, and integration of both order and energy, and it quickens the breath and excites the soul.

The ancient Greeks considered beauty a human need because, as Aristotle said, "no man can live without pleasure." He considered the pleasures we get from enjoying beauty to be higher pleasures, and when we are deprived of these, we "indulge excessively in the sensual pleasures."[44] When beauty stirs us emotionally we experience both esthetic and sensory pleasure.

FROM BASE PAIRS TO ALPINE TUNDRA

—no one can stand in these solitudes unmoved, and not feel that there is more in man than the mere breath of his body.

—DARWIN

Beauty, in the form of intrinsic elegance, clarity, and harmony, is a driving force for much science and, for theoretical physicists, is often used as a test of whether an equation is true.[45] When Francis Crick and James Watson finally put the base pairs together in a final model of the DNA molecule, a discovery that led to Nobel Prizes for them, they smiled and went out to lunch. They knew it was just too beautiful not to be right, "that a structure this pretty just had to exist."[46]

When I climb above timberline to peaks of 14,000 feet, I am breathless not only from the thin air but the beauty of "the land above the trees." A book by that name by Ann Zwinger and Beatrice Willard, expresses what I experience:

In the early morning the alpine tundra has a beginning-of-the-world quality, a sense of sparseness and lucidity. At high altitude, there is nothing between you and the sky; no tree branches, no filtering haze, no dulling pollution. Voices are often lost in the constant shushing of the wind. The tundra is a solitary world where one can feel very much alone and overwhelmed . . . a land of contrast and incredible intensity, where the sky is the size of forever and the flowers the size of a millisecond."[47]

The beauty of this world, I am convinced, did not happen by accident or happenstance. The world and its inhabitants could have evolved or been made without beauty, studies show.[48] "Plants can reproduce without flowers, as is indicated by many tons of coal formed of non-flowering plants some 345 million years ago. Not until 130 million years ago did flowering plants bloom as examples of nature's inherent impulse to emphasize beauty beyond strict necessity . . . while it is true that flowers exist to produce seeds, it is equally true that seeds exist to produce flowers. If nature produced humans concerned about beauty after survival was assured, why could not the rest of nature contain a similar impulse to produce beauty beyond the needs of reproduction?"[49]

Just as I delight in the carpets of dandelions across the mountain slopes as heralds of spring, I find great enjoyment in the beauty of aspen trees and their luminous tones of yellow and gold leaves as forerunners of fall. Only the aspen chooses to colonize "disturbed areas, such as roadsides or sites of forest fires or avalanches,"[50] which means it brings beauty to the barren, turning dross into gold.

HEALING GARDENS AT HOSPITALS

New feet within my garden go,
New fingers stir the sod . . .

—EMILY DICKINSON

Music, art, poetry, and literature—as well as mountains, seas, forests, flowers, lakes, and waterfalls—are healing. I think they heal by connecting us to a larger whole, which takes us out of our separate selves and joins us to a deeper, universal energy. They kindle our inner health and life force. They will not cure us of irreversible illnesses, but they will help us be well inside. Gardens have been found to soothe patients with cancer, Alzheimer's, and disabilities from strokes.[51] In California Topher Delaney, a garden designer, was herself diagnosed with breast cancer and, after being repelled by crowded waiting rooms and noisy cafeterias in hospital basements, she told herself: "Topher, you're going to spend the rest of whatever life you have making healing gardens." After Delaney underwent a mastectomy, she set out to build a garden in 800 square feet of outdoor space at the Marin General Hospital Cancer Center north of San Francisco. It has a stone fountain surrounded by such medicinal plants as echinacea, periwinkle, and yew. It is a quiet place for patients awaiting radiation and chemotherapy. Next, she was commissioned to build a two-acre meditation garden at the Norris Cancer Center in Los Angeles. She designed it for two different kinds of patients: Those "coming in who are panicked that they aren't going to survive" and "ones who aren't who are accepting it." In New York, at Howard A. Rusk Institution of Rehabilitation Medicine in Manhattan, a horticulture therapy program uses gardens in physical therapy. Said one patient regaining the use of her hands after a stroke: "It feels really good to be touching the soil and plants again."[52]

A REJUVENATING PLACE

All that in this delightful garden grows,
Should happy be, and have immortal bliss.

—SPENSER

Julie Moir Messervy believes that "deep within each of us lies a garden," an inward garden that we use as "both a sanctuary from the stress of everyday life and a place of rejuvenation."[53] She helps people design an outward garden, a landscape place that complements and reinforces their inward gardens. She quotes in her beautifully illustrated book, *The Inward Garden,* the Persian poet Rumi, who said that one's "outward spring and garden are the reflection of the inward garden."[54] Messervy learned the art of gardenmaking in Japan, where much emphasis is placed on creating spaces for opening the heart to "beauty and spirit." (See Chapter 7 for spiritual gardens and recovery from heart attacks).

Messervy found that gardens, both inner and outer, serve a number of psychological and physical functions, including healing. "A garden is as much a state of mind as it is an actual place. It exists because you discover a place of beauty that feels set apart in space and time."[55]

WHAT DAVID APPRECIATES

Appreciation of beauty is helping my schizophrenic son to heal, to find health within himself. Beauty has such power that it can even break through the most formidable disorders, as Dr. Oliver Sachs discovered with music and his post-encephalitis and Parkinsonism patients (see Chapter 3). My 37-year-old son has spent most of his adult life in mental hospitals. He has come from being locked up and shackled in maximum security wards—because he was violent—to living peacefully in a boarding home for discharged mental patients. He has profound appreciations, each one rooted in a deep sense of freedom.

The freedom David appreciates is not only the blessing of living outside the state hospital. It is a freedom that Clozaril, the first of a new generation of drugs for schizophrenia, has given him to appreciate the beauty of nature, the snow mantling city streets and sidewalks, covering the potholes and cracks, making even what is unsightly look fresh and new. David is now free to write about the beauty he sees, because Clozaril has given him freedom from being so preoccupied with paranoid thoughts and inner voices that he could not express himself except in anger. David now has the freedom to take pleasure in ordinary experiences, of walking, running, riding the bus. He is coming to know the freedom of giving and receiving love, of experiencing peace. On the wall of his small room he keeps posted a description he has written of his disease, of the voices he can still hear but not act on, of the feelings, less frequent now, that people are against him and talking about him, of the excessive dopamine in his brain from misfiring neurons and crossed-up nerve fibers. He feels free now to appreciate that even with such a disease, he has reason to be grateful for his life.

He has learned what powerful words *thank you* are. He says them freely now, and people respond. In his book, Miller, a psychologist, notes that saying "thank you" is a way to start having "conversations with God."[56] When we pray, we may petition and plead but we also express thanks and appreciation. David is beginning to do that.

When we regain a freedom to appreciate life again, powerful effects occur in the brain, even in the presence of existing disease. A tract of neurons and fibers that extend from the limbic system to the frontal lobes, with branches to other centers, carries our sense of being alive and the pleasure that conveys.[57] The tract, which is called the medial forebrain bundle[58] buzzes when we experience satisfaction in our very existence. I take pleasure in knowing that David's MFB is slowly rekindling. When he appreciates beauty, the MFB fires off a message in the brain and body that life is worth living.

SOMETHING MAX COULD APPRECIATE

Even when the brain and body are being invaded by metastatic cancer, appreciation of beauty can provide strong motivation to live. Four months before I met Maxine Olman she had been readmitted to M.D. Anderson Cancer Center and was told she had five days to live. "I was furious," she said, "that anyone had the audacity to tell me the days I had to live." Max had been a fighter even before she was first diagnosed in 1992 with metastatic ovarian cancer. She underwent three operations and high-dose chemotherapy and "dedicated myself to beating the sucker down so I could go back to my life." She participated in a cancer support group, she did guided imagery, music therapy, she joined a women's arts group, and she held a poetry writing class in her home and kept fighting. Finally, after a colostomy in the spring of 1995, she developed a systemic infection and signed up as a patient at The Hospice at the Texas Medical Center.

Max's social worker at the hospice told her: "You've spent most of your post-diagnosis time trying to convince yourself the glass is half full. Maybe it's time to spill the water out and concentrate on making the glass the most beautiful it can be." Max took this to mean it was time for her to shift from being angry and a fighter to recreating herself and her life into something beautiful. She said, "I had been brought up on the myth that when you're close to dying, what you will miss the most is something you never got to *do*. What suddenly hit me emotionally was that I had spent far too much of my life being angry and never satisfied with anything. I wanted now to *be* something different. Something I could appreciate."

Max became peaceful. She gave up fighting with her sister and father; she decided the best way to deal with her cancer was to make peace with it. Two weeks before she died, she did something I much admired and appreciated. Beautifully groomed and dressed, she stood before hospice staff and volunteers and gave a detailed, hour-long presentation on what it was like to be a patient there.[59] She expressed gratitude for what she had experienced as good and suggested corrections for what she saw as weaknesses. She spoke lovingly of her father, sitting nearby, and exchanged tears with those she felt closest to at hospice. Max had made her glass "the most beautiful it can be." Something she could appreciate.

MARY AND HER HUSBAND

Mary, 50, one of the women in our study, is the only one who lost a husband to cancer at the same time she was recovering from a modified radical mastectomy and 10 months of chemotherapy.[60] The beauty she appreciates in her life comes from the beach and the effects it had on both her husband and herself. Her husband's renal cell cancer, which had already metastasized by the time he was diagnosed, turned him into an angry, depressed, demanding person. She was beginning to "hate" him. But when Mary was diagnosed with breast cancer, he changed. They both started spending more and more time at their beach house in Galveston, looking at sunrises and sunsets, listening to the waves crashing on shore, hearing the sound of seagulls, focusing on the preciousness of life's moments. Their mutual anger turned to peace. Now, two and a half years after his death, Mary is making the beach house her full-time home. When she has to be away from it, she purposely keeps grains of sand in her shoes. "I want to keep mindful of that peace, that beauty."[61]

Chapter Six

MAKING OUR
PAIN SING

Alas for those who never sing,
But die with all their music in them.

—OLIVER WENDELL HOLMES

I f pain traps us inside ourselves, leaving no space for anything else in our lives, it would never seem to be a means by which we can discover a sense of greater wholeness and health. Yet people do use pain for such a discovery. Just as appreciation may bring us to a realization of well-being, pain can move us to a sense of being well inside ourselves that is larger than pain and trauma.

How does this transformation occur? A common denominator among the people I have known and worked with who have succeeded in using pain as a positive catalyst is this: They become so engaged in something outside themselves—something so completely self-absorbing—that pain becomes peripheral.

Pain is both a sensation and a perception.[1] The sensation of hurting is strongly affected by our perception of ourselves and our lives. The more we marvel at life and accept the challenges, good and bad, that it keeps throwing at us, the more opportunities we will see to lift ourselves outside of our pain.

JAMES HALL'S LOVE OF LIFE

The power of pain or trauma to trap us inside ourselves is more than a metaphor. A condition called the "locked-in syndrome" describes the position of a Dallas psychiatrist I know who suffered a brainstem stroke that left him without speech or the ability to move any part of his body. He could only blink his eyelids, which he did in answer to his doctor's question shortly after he suffered a stroke to the pons, a small area of the brain immediately above the spinal column. The doctor said: "Blink once for yes, twice for no. . . . Do you choose to live in this condition?" Doing all he could to make sure that he didn't involuntarily blink two times, "with all his might, James Hall blinked once. He chose life, no matter how difficult. He was 57 years old."[2]

What made the decision unequivocal for Hall was his fascination with life and the mind. He could still think, he could still probe into his own dreams and those of others (he's a Jungian psychiatrist), and after extensive physical rehabilitation, he could continue writing books, sitting in a wheelchair, and typing at a computer keyboard one letter at a time with a splint on one finger.

For an interviewer, he typed out, in the all capitals that he uses: "LIFE IS, IF ANYTHING, MORE INTERESTING THAN BEFORE I WAS DISABLED. I DON'T WORRY NOW ABOUT SUCH THINGS AS REPUTATION AND EARNING A LIVING. WITH ESSENTIALLY NOTHING TO LOSE, I AM MORE OPEN ABOUT WHAT I THINK."[3]

So Hall uses his mind to lift himself outside of the trauma that traps his body. By attaching himself to the thoughts that absorb him—God, analysis, fairy tales, dreams, what a person is—he loses himself and gains something greater: a kind of inner health and well-being he never had before. He writes:

"GOD, AS I CONCEIVE HIM/HER, COULD HEAL ME BUT WOULD NOT. IN A DEEP SENSE, THERE IS NOTHING TO 'HEAL' ME FROM. OBVIOUSLY COULD USE PHYSICAL HEALING TO RESTORE MY PREVIOUS LEVEL OF FUNCTION, BUT I AM PSYCHOLOGICALLY HEALTHIER THAN I HAVE EVER BEEN."

A Butterfly's Way Out

. . . the mature imagination of a man is healthy.

—KEATS

Like James Hall, Jean-Dominique Bauby, a 44-year-old French magazine editor and father of two young children, suffered a catastrophic stroke that left him without movement or speech and required him to rely solely on his nonphysical self to rise above his continued pain and corporeal confinement.[4] Also a victim of locked-in syndrome, Bauby devised a communication system based on blinking that permitted him to "dictate" a book one letter at a time. He produced a moving memoir using only his left eyelid to signal which letter he wanted to be written down from a rearranged alphabet.

His book, *Le Scaphandre et le Papillon* (The Diving Bell and the Butterfly), describes how Bauby's rich imagination permitted him to take flight out of his physical prison. He said, "my mind takes flight like a butterfly. There is so much to do. You can wander off in space or in time, set out for Tierra del Fuego or for King Midas' court" or, vicariously, "sit down to a meal at any hour with no fuss or ceremony. . . . If I do the cooking, it's always a success."[5] Bauby doesn't hide his despair but he makes an art of using pain to create beauty. At the end of his 132 pages, he asks, "Does the cosmos keep keys for opening up my diving bell? . . . We must keep looking?" Two days after his book was published to wide acclaim in France, his search ended. Bauby died suddenly, leaving behind a marvelous record of a spirit that soared.

THE MYTH OF TWO PAINS

Initially, when trauma and pain strike, we may find mixed with the fear about what will happen to us a great deal of anger that it happened in the first place. The anger may be at God for letting it happen, at ourselves for somehow not avoiding it, at individuals in our lives, past and present, who have hurt us badly, or at all the healthy people we know who seem to deserve pain more than we do. Our anger may energize us for awhile, but over time it keeps us self-focused and trapped within our pain.

Mary, the real estate agent whose husband was in the hospital with metastatic cancer at the same time she was being treated for breast cancer, was so mad at God she stopped going to the synagogue and told her rabbi she wasn't coming back. Two other women in our study told me of rage at their fathers for having incestuous relations with them as children and denying it ever happened. When we have a serious illness and are lying flat on our backs day after day, anger and despair easily well up from the past and compound the pain of the present. "Our pain...is layered with our unique memories, emotions and thoughts," research shows.[6] Because "pain states" can exist as a "reliving of past pain experience" and be just as real as a broken bone or tissue damage,[7] the more we let the past go, the less our pain will be.

Dr. David B. Morris, whose career has centered on researching pain and helping people manage it, emphasizes that "the myth of two pains," one mental and one physical, is untrue. The reality is that the mental, emotional, and physical constantly interact, each affecting the other and giving us one total experience of pain. When we hurt emotionally, it affects us physically. When we hurt physically, it affects us emotionally.[8] As to two other types of pain, acute and chronic, they too can come together as one. Most people, with their doctors, "eventually figure out how to handle acute pain, which comes after injuries or surgeries" or advanced stages of diseases like cancer.⁹ "But nothing prepares us for chronic pain," which saps our vitality and drains our savings. Because pain is so multi-layered, coming out of and feeding on so many facets of our lives, our relationships and attitudes, what begins as acute pain often becomes chronic pain.

MARY'S SOLUTION

For it is in giving that we receive....

—ST. FRANCIS OF ASSISI

So it takes something powerful to make pain peripheral to our lives. No drug can do it or, at least, keep doing it. Mary permanently gave up the question, "Why me?" and her anger at God when her cancer led her to the discovery of a creative gift so engrossing she came out of herself. After losing her hair from chemotherapy and trying to find scarves for her head that were attractive, she began experimenting with her own designs and novel ways of tying the material.

Mary found she has a marvelous gift for design and fashion, and her scarves have become a passion with her. She enlisted her housekeeper, a black woman who learned as a child all the best ways to knot, tie, and wear scarves, and a friend to join her in starting a program teaching patients to "look better, feel better" from the scarves they wear and the make-up they apply during treatment and its aftermath. Mary sees her gift as "God-given" and coming directly out of her painful experience with cancer. Between being caught up in her "look better, feel better" program and love for her beach house, her life now is outside of pain. "I wake up each day, thinking this is a new day, and I'm going to enjoy every minute of it." She feels deep satisfaction from the improvement in morale and spirit that her program makes in the lives of fellow cancer survivors she works with.

Doing something of service to others is a creative response to pain that helps us hurt less. The evidence suggests that altruism is associated with having fewer episodes of illness and living longer.[10] When we truly invest ourselves in helping others we put our own pain to beneficial use. The cancer patients I interview often tell me that if their stories or experience can help someone else or contribute to research, they are glad to spend time talking with me.

THE POWER OF SERVICE

The measure of a life, after all,
is not its duration but its donation.

—PETER MARSHALL

Many cancer survivors do volunteer work at hospitals and cancer centers. The University of Texas M.D. Anderson Cancer Center has a huge network, run by volunteers, that offers a wide range of activities and programs, including a national annual conference that attracts thousands of patients and ex-patients from all over the world. Much of the work of volunteers is one-on-one support and encouragement for the newly diagnosed.

Betty's rheumatoid arthritis was so painful she was spending more and more days at home alone in bed. Then she received a desperate call from a lifelong, close friend, whose son, Larry, was at hospice with renal and liver failure and not expected to live much longer. Her friend asked Betty if she would come sit during the day with Larry and let him know someone who knew and loved him was with him. Larry's parents sat with him at night and on weekends but had to work during the day to keep money coming in. Betty had doubts that she was physically able to get to hospice but she couldn't turn her friend down, particularly because she had known Larry since being present at his birth.

The next day, with many trepidations, she somehow managed to drive herself to hospice and spent the day with Larry. Each day it got easier. Each day she surprised herself more. What she found incredible was that her deep arthritic pain had left her. She was walking everywhere without hurting and it was wonderful. "I guess God was telling me that I had to help someone else to help myself. I needed to serve in order to heal."

As is true of many of the wounded well in this book, they quietly take on some kind of service after they have worked through some of their own pain, anger, or grief —or even in the midst of it. Rachel Naomi Remen (Chapter 4) remembers a patient whose real recovery started when he decided one day to help others. "I had a man in my practice with osteogenic sarcoma of the leg, which was removed at the hip in order to save his life. He was 21 years old when I started working with him and he was a very angry man with a lot of bitterness, a deep sense of injustice and very deep hatred for all the well people because it seemed so unfair to him that he had suffered this terrible loss so early in life."[11]

But the young man gradually mustered the courage to change. He began "coming out of himself" after a couple of years. He started visiting other people in the hospital who had sustained severe physical losses "and he would tell me," Remen said, "the most wonderful stories about these visits." One was with a young woman about his age whose cancer treatment included removal of both breasts. It was "a hot day in Palo Alto and he was in running shorts so his artificial leg showed when he came into her hospital room." The woman was so depressed she would not even look at him.

The nurses had left her radio playing probably in order to cheer her up. So, desperate to get her attention, he unstrapped his leg and began dancing around the room on one leg, snapping his fingers to the music. She looked at him in amazement, and then she burst out laughing and said, "Man, if you can dance, I can sing."[12]

STRONG AT THE "BROKEN PLACES"

When the young man was ready to leave therapy with Remen, she pulled out the drawings he had done two years earlier in treatment. One was a picture of his body in the form of a vase with a deep black crack running through it. He was "grinding his teeth with rage at the time . . . . It seemed this vase could never function as a vase again."[13] The young man now remarked, "this one isn't finished," and he put his finger on the crack and said, "You see, this is where the light comes through." He then took a yellow crayon and drew light "streaming through the crack in his body." Remen knows "we can grow strong at the broken places" because she not only has seen her patients do it but she also has learned strength from her own pain. She has had Crohn's disease for 35 years, including major surgery seven times.

Using pain to bring benefit or pleasure to others has long served as a strong motivation for artists and writers. One of Georgia O'Keefe's early charcoal drawings is of a headache. "It was a very bad headache at the time that I was busy drawing every night, sitting on the floor in front of the closet door," she said. "Well, I had the headache, why not do something with it?" she thought. So she set out to make it into a work of art.[14] Morris observes that "at the extreme limit of art's transforming power . . . we might say that such pain becomes, no matter how improbable the thought, not merely an occasion for art but even a possible source of beauty."

When we are able to create something beautiful that gives pleasure to others, we are doubly blessed. Pain diminishes in direct proportion to what we give of ourselves that enriches people's lives. Arthur Fiedler, longtime conductor of the Boston Pops, had severe chronic asthma all the years he entertained television audiences and the thousands who went to his concerts at Symphony Hall or the Bandshell on the Charles River.[15]

Fiedler's energy and love for music remained undiminished by advancing years. The public was largely unaware that he suffered a chronic disorder. Backstage at intermission, Fiedler would cough and wheeze uncontrollably as he took medicine and tried to take a full, deep breath. Those present would swear he could never continue the program. Yet as soon as curtain time came, he straightened up, the coughing and wheezing stopped, and he stepped on stage as lively as ever. He connected to a higher register that lifted him out of his pain.

MAKING PAIN SING

Pain makes men think.

—JOHN PATRICK

The "singers" in Navaho healing practices of the Dineh, the largest tribe in North America, a herding people who have lived in the southwestern United States for centuries, are healers who conduct ceremonies that last from two to nine days and nights.[16] Those with pain and illness and many others in their community attend, since just to be present is considered healing. The "sings" and "chants" they hear date back centuries and even a single one requires several years for the healers to learn. In making pain sing, the ceremony is restorative in that it gives social support to the sick and integrates them back into the community.

Writers and poets have long made pain sing in other ways—by using it to make literature that moves us in mind, body, and spirit. Ernest Hemingway, whose tough-guy credo failed him in the end, said of pain, "We are all bitched from the start and you especially have to be hurt like hell before you can write seriously. But when you get the damned hurt use it—don't cheat with it. Be as faithful to it as a scientist."[17] Hemingway stopped using the pain in his own life in his final depression, which resulted in his suicide in 1961.

Gerry Coffee, the former POW in Chapter 3 whose motto was "Unity over Self," began his long confinement in North Vietnam with prayers asking "Why me, God?"[18] They slowly changed to "Show me, God, how to use this experience," as he saw ways to turn his suffering into something of value.

John Keats, a much earlier romantic counterpart to Hemingway's tough-guy realism, transformed his pain into poetry. Rita and I made a point to visit the stately house at the foot of the Spanish Steps in Rome, where Keats died. I read Keats because of his relentless quest for beauty and his conviction, which he held to the very end, that it is truth. It gives me pleasure to know that 200 years after Keats' birth, scholars and lovers of his poetry still gather at conferences to honor his life and writings, as they did in 1995 at Harvard.[19] Keats wrote his finest poems during the three years before his death when he was struggling hardest. For much of 1818 he nursed his brother Tom, who died in his arms of tuberculosis. By the end of that year, Keats suspected he had the disease himself. His mother had died of TB when he was 10. His first publication of poetry received a devastating reception from the London critics, who considered him callow and oversensitive. Financial worries beset him. He was depressed and considered giving up writing. Then he met and fell in love with Fanny Brawne, but it was "a hopeless passion in view of his poverty and illness."[20]

Although Keats had been panned for writing, "A thing of beauty is a joy forever:/Its loveliness increases,"[21] he stood by an aesthetic creed that insists that there is "something of the timeless and the deathless" in beauty.[22] Fanny Brawne nursed him during the winter of 1820 when a diagnosis of tuberculosis became definite. She would slip notes under Keats' door each night expressing her love. But by the next summer, after his condition had grown worse and she had been discouraged from seeing him, the poet left with the painter Joseph Severn for Italy, thanks to Keats' publisher raising necessary funds among his friends. In Rome Keats and Severn rented rooms in the four-story house close by the Barcaccia fountain and Spanish Steps. Severn wrote that Keats showed "no fear of death, no want of fortitude."[23]

Rita and I went to the English cemetery in Rome where Keats is buried. On his tombstone are the words he asked Severn to use as his epitaph three days before he died: "Here lies one whose name was writ on water." Although the words are from Sophocles, Severn believed Keats was also thinking of the endless sound of water he heard from the Barcaccia fountain outside their rooms. It seemed to dissolve his pain and carry him beyond it. Keats knew how to find beauty as darkness comes, as he said in his ode *To Autumn*: "Where are the songs of Spring? Ay, where are they?/ Think not of them, thou hast thy music too—."[24]

COURAGE TO CHANGE OURSELVES

Often the test of courage is not to die but to live.
—ALFIERI

Changing ourselves so that we hear music when we have a pain that has no cure may not be so much a matter of writing poetry as having the courage to change our lives. When Reinhold Niebuhr wrote the prayer in 1943 known today as *The Serenity Prayer,* he asked God to give us the strength to bear the things that cannot be changed, the courage to change what can and should be changed, and the wisdom to know the difference. The changes we need to make in ourselves are the hardest, Niebuhr believed. Some pain cannot be changed, but how we respond to it can if we have the courage to change ourselves.

The pain of cancer stays with survivors in the ever-present threat of recurrence. The women in our study who seem to be coping the best have shown the courage to make deep changes in their lives. They have stopped trying to be everything to everyone, never saying no, always pleasing, always trying to do more, accumulating more materially. They have started practicing paying attention to the birds, the bees, to flowers and trees and the good, green earth, and to the great value of having a God and people who love them. The changes have not come easily, but they are a powerful part of their having a sense of health.

Several years ago I was told at a free screening for prostate cancer that I needed to have further tests, including an ultrasound examination and a biopsy. The ultrasound showed an abnormal prostate but the biopsy did not show cancer. I was told to undergo retesting in three months. Meanwhile, my depression deepened over our daughter whose heart had been severely damaged by drugs but who kept using them, making her death inevitable. Despite antidepressants and therapy, I worried that my depression would suppress my immune system and tip the balance in my abnormal prostate toward cancer.

I slowly gathered the courage to change. I stopped hiding Liz's plight from others, I went to Twelve-Step support groups, and openly declared my pain and hers. I prayed more and attended chapel at the hospital across the street from my office during the week. And finally, just as spring began, I started reading *The Tibetan*

Book of the Living and Dying, but it was slow going and torturous for me. I was still not ready to accept death as part of life. Then I attended the seminar on death and dying by the surgeon who saw it as a cause to celebrate life, and I slowly stopped running from mortality, Liz's and my own. My depression began to lift, I could hear music again, I saw the beauty in art, I went to the mountains, and I waited for our daughter to die, but now I was responding differently to the pain. On my prostate retest, my PSA was lower, my prostate still felt and looked abnormal to my examiners, but the biopsy was still negative, and I felt blessed.

DEPRESSION AND PAIN

At the end of the mind, the body.
But at the end of the body, the mind.

—PAUL AMBROISE VALÉRY

My longtime acquaintance with pain began when I was a 24-year-old newspaper reporter, and I was assigned to go on the train with a group of railroad retirees taking a long "busman's holiday" to El Paso, Texas, and Juarez, Mexico. I returned with a bad case of diarrhea. After tests showed no sign of amoebic dysentery or other complications, I thought my belly would stop hurting. But it didn't. I continued to work but went from doctor to doctor, having more tests done (all negative) and seeking relief (none forthcoming). I finally took sick leave and went to a noted psychiatrist who specialized in psychosomatic disorders. I saw him every day for a week in psychotherapy, the aching in my gut unrelieved. He told me he had only one other recommendation: electroshock therapy. He never said I was depressed, and I didn't want to believe it. I decided to leave without any EST, but I later had to admit my depression when all the classic symptoms overtook me: loss of pleasure in life, loss of interest in most everything, chronic fatigue, inability to make decisions, lack of appetite, and withdrawl from others. The deeper the depression went, the less I cared about anything, even the aching in my belly. This became the pattern for each episode of the illness I have had since then. There have been no episodes in the last few years, but the pain has never completely left. So I try to put it to good use and make it sing.

What Gay Has Learned About Pain

My friend and colleague, Gay Robertson, knows more about making pain literally sing than anyone else I know. She has been a singer and musician since the age of 10, concentrating as an adult on oratorios and operas. "Without music I am absolutely convinced I would not have survived the experiences of my life," she said.[25] Those experiences include a childhood of physical, sexual, and emotional abuse, a pulmonary embolism with serious lung complications that nearly killed her after the birth of her first child, a triple coronary artery bypass operation at age 54, and life-threatening coronary problems since, which continue to send her to the hospital for angioplasty and more medication.

"I don't sing," Gay says, "because I love it (although I do). I sing because I must! If I don't sing, I can't breathe. Performing is not particularly important to me; but music is my soul, and singing is the connection between my inner being, my physical self, and the outside world. Without it, all my life experience is locked away and useless."

What Gay's life experience has taught her about pain is not to fear it. The blood clot in the lung after the birth of her first child she remembers as the most physically painful time of her life. "I learned that even though I would like to have howled and screamed, I couldn't afford the air, and though I wanted to cry, that made it impossible to breathe. One *can* learn to deal with intense pain, as well as with fear, and can ultimately achieve almost a form of transcendence. You can find a place of peace and calm deep inside where you can ride atop the waves of pain and fear. To learn these things early gives a person a very useful tool for the rest of their life."

Gay brings to her singing an understanding of life and pain that gives a richer meaning to the music. I have never asked her if she had her life to live over, how much of the pain would she want cut out of it. "People who most fear pain," she believes, "are those who have experienced very little of it . . . . Those people who have experienced great pain, particularly prolonged pain, and especially pain associated with a life-threatening injury or illness, go through various stages, winding up seeing pain as their companion, fighting the illness together, coping with what life throws at them, and forcing them into plumbing the depths and heights of their soul and capacities."

Because the total experience of pain is fed by multiple streams of distress, some physical, some psychological, it diminishes when we do the hard work of clearing up log jams and debris in our lives. Gay had to make peace with the people in her family, now gone, who abused her from the time she was 1 year old. Years of psychotherapy helped her do this.

PAST SEXUAL ABUSE, PRESENT PAIN

I had no time to hate, because

The grave would hinder me,

And life was not so ample I

Could finish enmity.

—EMILY DICKINSON

Dorothy, the cancer survivor with Crohn's disease, was sexually abused by her father from age 3 to 12.[26] She didn't recognize what a damaging and depressing effect it was having on her life until she was in her 30s and went into therapy for two years. But it was not until after she had her mastectomy that she read one day about another woman who got breast cancer and was described by Bernie Siegel as needing "to get things off her chest." That hit home with her. Her father had always told her never to tell her mother about the incest because it would "destroy her." Dorothy phoned her mother and told her in great anger what had happened all those years. She was angry that her mother, now long divorced from Dorothy's father, had not protected her. Instead of being destroyed, her mother listened sympathetically and became supportive. Dorothy went to Washington and had a face-to-face confrontation with her father. He denied the incest ever happened. Even if it did, he said, he couldn't believe it would have such an effect on her life. "You always seem so successful," he'd say. She decided he was a sociopath.

The confrontation relieved some of the pain but not all. Later, she "cried and cried" on the phone to her father, sobbing "this is how I feel. Can you understand?" Still, there was pain left. Another call, this time in a rage. "I yelled and yelled at him, so much so he put his wife—my stepmother—on the phone to hear it." Her father eventually acknowledged in a halfhearted way that the incest may have occurred. But by then, Dorothy didn't need the admission. The pain was off her chest.

Ellen, a 50-year-old nurse who had a lumpectomy and radiation after her mammogram detected a tumor in late 1993, has slowly let go of resentment toward her father, now dead, who sexually abused her.[27] She too has had long-term psychotherapy for depression. Fifteen years after his death, she planned the first trip ever to her father's grave in Philadelphia. "I have not forgotten what happened, but I have forgiven him."

━━━━━━━━━━━━━

LILLY AND FORGIVING

A wise man will make haste to forgive,
because he knows the true value of time.

—SAMUEL JOHNSON

Forgiving is another way to lessen the pain in our lives. But we forgive slowly when we have been deeply hurt or betrayed. Pain may push us toward forgiveness when it comes from the knowledge that we may die soon and we want to wash clean the angers and resentments that our life has accumulated. Lilly (Chapter 3) decided after a recurrence of her cancer that she didn't want to die hating anyone or having anyone hate her. She concluded she needed to have forgiving talks with four people in her life. She called them and either asked their forgiveness or said she forgave them. In all four cases, there was much relief on both sides. "It was the most freeing thing to do," she said, "and it cost me nothing."

Letting go of the ego is a prerequisite to forgiveness and often occurs when we don't know how much time we have left to live. "Carrying baggage from the past only hurts you," Lilly said. "I don't want to leave this world having unfinished business."[28]

The hardest forgiving Lilly had to do was of her own husband, who had had an affair with her best friend, who was also on her forgiveness list. To forgive, Lilly says, "you have to get to the point where you see that some things don't have anything to do with you." She decided to stay with her husband and has not regretted the decision. He is now very caring and supportive. Lilly is "positive and upbeat" and wants to live "for as long as I can the best I can."

Grief, as much as betrayal and physical trauma, leaves holes left to fill. After the death of her grandmother Rose, Marlee Matlin, winner of an Academy Award for her portrayal of a deaf student in *Children of a Lesser God,* could not comprehend "a day without her gentle smile and caring touch. The loss was so painful. But as days and months passed, I found that the pain I felt began to transform itself into something completely new. The empty hole in my life was slowly filled in with a warmth." She would remember her grandmother's words of encouragement and began "to understand that my successes and achievements were her pats on the back, her hugs when I was discouraged and her stories of her dreams and hopes for her children and grandchildren when I had none." Then it became clear that "my life was an extension of hers. When there is a hole someplace in the world, I believe a warmth eventually fills it. When there is poverty, a richness of spirit eventually comes to help. I believe we are here for each other; to lift, to encourage, to dream. Without that kind of giving we cease to exist . . . ."[29]

How Humor Helps

Laughter is the closest thing to the grace of God.

—KARL BARTH

We would also cease to exist, to bear pain and make it useful, without laughter. When Deanna, barely 40, came to the final realization she was losing her hair from chemotherapy, she broke down in heavy sobbing.[30] Even a gentle pull brought hair out by the handful. After weeping inconsolably, she began playing games of making streaks in her hair by pulling more of it out. Then she opened her bedroom door and called to her teenage daughter to come see. The mother asked the daughter how she liked her new hairstyle and invited her to join in the game. Together they made streaks until all her hair was gone. And they laughed to the very end.

Sandy was so depressed from getting cancer, having her husband leave her, and being without a job, she wanted to die and went to surgery with that wish in mind.[31] She had read that we see light upon dying, so when she began seeing light after being put to sleep, she thought she had died. "But what I was seeing were the fluorescent lights in my hospital room after surgery. I could only laugh about it and still do. My kids don't think it's that funny, but it helps me to lighten up."

Chapter Seven

LIVING

WITH

PURPOSE

Meaningless inhibits fullness of life
and is therefore equivalent to illness.
Meaning makes a great many things endurable
—perhaps everything.

—JUNG

For many of the wounded but well, the sick or impaired who have discovered a different kind of health, the most powerful use of pain is to find purpose and meaning in it. When we do that, we not only suffer less, we also discover a new way to live well.

The power of purpose can not only lift us above the sharp pain of an injury or acute illness but see us through the dark tunnel of depression or progressive infirmity. Sometimes the best purpose we can put pain and illness to is letting others see that it is possible to overcome even the disease that kills us.

Nelson Butters did that. Those who were with Butters as he went from being a vibrant teacher and researcher at Johns Hopkins to degenerating physically for three long years because of Lou Gehrig's disease were "struck by how he overcame the disease by staying purposeful, lively, and wittily intelligent right through to the end, teaching much to all of us."[1] In prevailing over his disease in spirit, if not physically, Butters, who was 58 when he died, taught his fellow faculty members, physicians, and friends how powerful a dedication to life can be—even to just a spark of life, which was all he had left at the end.

Each time he had to surrender more of his body to the disease—"accepting a wheelchair, retreating to bed, undergoing a tracheostomy to facilitate breathing"—he would become despondent for a time but "he recovered his cheer as he found himself more comfortable and able to continue his work with students and colleagues and his life with his family."[2] Toward the end he used computers, as Stephen Hawking does, to communicate and work.

THREE MAJOR GAINS

Butters edited a major journal in neuropsychology, his specialty, "even when he could move only one finger and then only one toe. With these small movements he used e-mail to write to colleagues everywhere—usually on professional matters, but also to transmit amusing academic gossip."[3] When the only strength he had left was the ability to blink his eyes, he gathered his family around him, and had his doctors turn off the ventilator that breathed for him. He soon slipped into a coma and died.

His friend, Dr. Paul R. McHugh, the Henry Phipps professor and director of psychiatry and behavioral sciences at Hopkins, said that by "permitting a progressive infirmity to continue right out to its natural end," Butters scored three major gains in the face of death. He continued his work as a scientist, editor, and teacher for many months. He extended the time he had with his wife and children, "no trivial matter, for he was a lovable person."[4] From the experience of helping to nurse him, one of his daughters decided to take up a career in nursing incapacitated persons. Last, he made the doctors who helped him at each stage to withstand his physical degeneration feel appreciated and proud as Butters took what they offered "and made more of it."

HELPING OTHERS IS THE HIGHEST MEANING

Give, and it shall be given unto you

is still the truth about life.

—D. H. LAWRENCE

Being of service, which Butters was to the very end, consists of committing ourselves to something bigger than the self, and it provides dramatic proof of how meaning and purpose transcend suffering. Viktor Frankl, who lived more than 50 years afterward, learned in the Nazi death camps that "to use your suffering to help others is . . . the highest of all meanings."[5]

Soldiers who strongly believe in the purpose of the war they are fighting often feel little or no pain when wounded. They use "neutral terms like 'bang' and 'thump' to describe losing a limb."[6] The purpose of an athlete is to win, and the focus required often keeps the pain from being admitted to awareness. A ballet dancer accepts pain as part of the price of superb performance from endless hours of practice and self-discipline. In fact, "pain is the unchosen but inevitable medium of performance."[7]

For all of us, life in a sense is a performance. We respond to roles and events—some are chosen, many are not—and pain, whether physical, psychological, or both, finds its way into many of them. But when we have a larger purpose in life, we "have something better to do," and we don't suffer as much, as Fordyce's law promises.[8] We may hurt, we may endure long, dark nights of the soul, but we avoid becoming victims by a deep attachment to a goal. If we are in remission, then we should use the word to remind us to *regenerate* a *mission*.

PURPOSE STRONGER THAN PAIN

What can a meaning outside my condition mean to me? I can understand only in human terms. What I touch, what resists—that is what I understand.

—CAMUS

How do we do that? How do we come by a purpose that is stronger than pain? Psychologist and clinical researcher Martin Seligman is convinced that finding meaning requires "an attachment to something larger than oneself. And the larger the entity, the more meaning there is to be derived. To the extent that it is now difficult for young people to take seriously their relationship with God, to care about their relationship with the country, or to be part of a large and abiding family, meaning in life will be very difficult to find. The self, to put it another way, is a very poor site for meaning."[9] If we reach beyond the self for larger identities, we expand our consciousness and get a different view of our pain, our problems. Psychologist/physician Carl Jung (see Chapter 4) made this observation:

> ...I have often seen individuals simply outgrow a problem which had destroyed others. This "outgrowing"... was seen to consist in a new level of consciousness. Some higher or wider interest arose on the person's horizon, and through this widening of his view the insoluble problem lost its urgency.[10]

DEANNA CAME OUT OF HERSELF

To be a whole person we must

get ourselves off our hands.

—FOSDICK

Some twenty years ago, when Deanna (see Chapter 6) gave birth to her first child, a baby boy badly crippled by cerebral palsy and retarded, she was devastated. She wept long and hard and became depressed. Then she became angry and determined. She began to see a purpose in what had happened to her. It was to teach her to recognize and use her inner strength, to use pain not to contract her life but to expand it—to reach out to others, to stop being a loner and self-absorbed. All of her life she had been shy and quiet, spending much time by herself. Now she was called to be a fighter. "They didn't expect him to live, much less walk, talk, learn shapes, colors." Not only did her son live, "he learned to walk, talk, read, and will graduate from high school next year" at age 21. It would never have happened if she had not discovered she had the strength to make it happen. Schools wouldn't take her son, doctors were pessimistic about his ever developing. She had to be aggressive and a fighter to get him the help and resources that have brought him to where he is today. The painful experience of having a handicapped child "turned my life around," she believes. In seeing that the purpose was to get her out of herself, she found more health in herself.

Deanna not only tapped her hidden reservoir of internal power to provide her son with what he needed but she also used it to raise a daughter, three years younger than her son, to survive a divorce, and to build a career as a computer systems specialist for a large corporation. Then she got cancer. She could have asked, "Why me, haven't I already had enough pain?" But she didn't. She could have believed God was punishing her, but she didn't, because "my God wouldn't do that." She saw her cancer as just another test of inner strength. Her new resolve was to stay alive in order to assure that her son would get the care he needed and that she could raise her daughter into adulthood. After a modified radical mastectomy she had chemotherapy that made her so sick she has questioned whether she would ever submit to such treatment again if she had a recurrence. "I decided I would." Her purpose was to be here for her children, particularly her disabled son.

But now that, for the first time, her son is happily living in a group home, Deanna has a new purpose that sustains her. She keeps before her an image of the green countryside of Tennessee at the foot of the Cumberland Mountains. "You can feel it, smell it, it is beautiful. Everything is green." This is her "meditation place," the scene she images when she meditates and the one she used in the imagery group of our breast cancer project. Deanna grew up in Tennessee, and she particularly remembers her grandparents' place in Westchester near the mountains. She lived there once for a while when she was married. Now she wants to return for good. "It's home, where my roots are." She will be returning to nature, because one part of her image has her gardening and being outdoors more. "I want a bigger garden than now, one where I can grow vegetables to cook and can."

AN ANSWER TO "WHY ME?"

If I can stop one heart from breaking,

I shall not live in vain;

If I can ease one life the aching,

or cool one pain,

or help one fainting robin

Unto his nest again,

I shall not live in vain.

—EMILY DICKINSON

Purpose is so powerful because it gives us reason to live and concrete goals to achieve. It organizes, energizes, and directs us. It has been said that "the ultimate in well-being is to have all of one's life flowing toward an overriding goal, a unifying life theme, that gives meaning to all our lesser goals."[11] Most of us settle for a series of lesser goals, but if we examine them closely, we often find an underlying theme and purpose.

In pain, purpose gives us an answer to "Why me?" The mother of a critically ill baby born prematurely said: "We know that seven out of every 100 babies are born prematurely. We know that a problem with my uterus was the cause. But that doesn't help me answer the question, 'Why us and not someone else?' "[12]

Researchers have found that mothers like this one commonly conclude that "God has a plan for them" or that their crisis is "a test of their faith." Still others see themselves as "privileged to have been chosen to be the parent of a child with special needs."[13] Their purpose becomes the honoring of that privilege.

The evidence from one study shows that "those who were able to find some purpose in this event" before their baby was discharged from the newborn intensive care unit "displayed greater responsiveness to their child's needs in the first months of caring for their child at home."[14]

Purpose, to be stronger than pain, has to be attached to deeply fulfilling goals, that is, to goals that are true ends and not just means to an end. Ends satisfy us so that when we reach them, we don't ask, "Is this all there is?" Accumulating possessions, power, popularity, and prestige, does not pass the true-ends test. There is always "something more" we are hungry for and it can't be satisfied by material success. It does not satisfy the spirit or keep us well inside ourselves. Studies show that a sense of well-being is not correlated with how much money or status we have.[15] It is correlated with love, faith, and courage—and, I would add, beauty.

REDUCING RISK OF RECURRENCE

Researchers have found that people recovering from a serious myocardial infarction who are willing to open their hearts to more love often reduce their risks of having another heart attack, which often kills them.[16] Recognizing that the purpose of their heart attack was to sound an alarm bell signaling the need to change their lives becomes a major motivator. What most of these men and women find they must do is to change lifelong priorities that have made material success their god and to cultivate their "spiritual part."[17] Many of them score high on time-urgency, impatience, and cynicism or hostility, which makes change that much harder.

Dr. Carl Thoresen of Stanford, a psychologist on the Recurrent Coronary Prevention Project at Mount Zion Hospital in San

Francisco, considers "spirit" to be neither abstract nor necessarily religious; it is very physical and basic—it means "breath" in the widest and most literal sense.[18] "Spiritual" is anything that promotes breathing, feeling alive, living fully. Pain is often what leads us to discovering our spiritual part and recognizing that an important source of breath is love. Those who plant a "spiritual garden," as Thoresen calls it, place new importance on family and friends, music, prayer, and less on "I," "mine," and "me." (See Chapter 5 for other inward gardens).

Research has shown that excessive self-involvement, as measured by frequency counts of personal references, predicts risk of coronary occlusions.[19] When Sociologist Robert Bellah of the University of California at Berkeley wrote *Habits of the Heart,* he interviewed people considered successes, "the cream of the crop," and found they could talk only about self, with little sense of community.[20] In closing the heart and shutting out others, we deny our spiritual part, which gives breath and sparks our inner health.

Physical health as well as subjective well-being is enhanced by opening the heart, as confirmed by controlled, follow-up studies of both the Recurrent Coronary Prevention Project and Dr. Dean Ornish's studies.[21] Similar results have been reported from the Army War College, where top officers at risk of cardiovascular disease and heart attacks were put in a "change" program. Those who did change not only became healthier and more productive for the Army, they became more loved by their families.[22]

MEANINGS WE GIVE TO ILLNESS

Hold every moment sacred.
Give each clarity and meaning,
each the weight of thine awareness . . . .

—MANN

The meaning we give to our illness or disability, our heart attack or cancer or paralysis, is as important as the purpose we create for our lives. If we tell ourselves that the meaning of our myocardial infarction or cancer recurrence is that we will never be able to work again, we will suffer physiologically as well as psychologically. Dossey admitted a man to a coronary care unit with intense chest pain, and tests were begun to determine whether he had suffered a heart attack.[23]

After the pain diminished, he lay on his bed and studied the cardiac monitor he was wired up to. He noticed that the oscilloscope registered a steady heart rate of about 80 per minute. In the next 24 hours, the patient found that he could have a significant effect on his heart rate by the meaning he attached to his chest pain. He could make his heart rate settle in the 60s or climb slowly to the 90s. "If I want my heart rate to fall, I close my eyes and focus on the chest pain. I let it *mean* to me that it's only indigestion or perhaps muscle pain. I know it's nothing; I'll be back at work tomorrow. If I want to increase the heart rate, I switch the meaning. I think the worst: I've had a real heart attack. I'll never get back to work. I'm just waiting around for the big one."[24] The man's tests showed he had not had an MI after all, so his more benign meaning proved accurate.

What meaning we attach to our illness is powerfully shaped by how mindful we are that in every circumstance, even the most adverse, there is some value to be found, some benefit, some gift. We don't have to be Pollyannish to be mindful, simply aware that we have a choice to read either dire meanings of darkness into a situation or something more bright and hopeful. Which we choose will contribute to the outcome.

GROWING SPIRIT AND COURAGE

Illness often means change, either good or bad. Change, particularly for those whose success in life has brought them not only material affluence but recognition from others, takes courage. "Courage" comes from the heart. The word is related to the French *coeur,* and to the Latin *cor* and *coraticum.*[25] It refers to the seat of our spirit, as Shakespeare knew when he had Queen Margaret say to Henry: "...this soft courage makes your followers faint,"[26] referring to weak spirit. Courage is critical to reconnecting to our core, our ground of being, our sense of wholeness. If we plant thymos—which stands for the courageous element of the soul[27]—in our spiritual gardens, we should grow spirit. It relates to the "middle" of a person's being, theologian Paul Tillich said, and gives us an "unreflective striving toward what is noble."[28] "Courage is the affirmation of one's essential nature, one's inner aim...."[29] It is necessary for those with prolonged or recurring illness to find and cultivate.

"Thymos"—courage—has been associated with healing in more than a metaphorical sense. Thyme, whose name is related to thymos, was found to be a herb with medicinal and antibiotic powers. The thymus gland, at the base of the throat, plays an important role in the immune system and etymologically comes from the same root as thyme and thymos.

What Jung would have us pay attention to in our spiritual gardens is rhizome, a rich root system, characteristic of such flowers as irises, which spreads horizontally making myriad connections underground. Jung saw rhizome as our collective unconscious, our connection to God. His view:

> Life has always seemed to me like a plant that lives on its rhizome. Its true life is invisible, hidden in the rhizome. The part that appears above ground lasts only a single summer. . . . I have never lost a sense of something that lives and endures underneath the eternal flux. What we see is the blossom, which passes. The rhizome remains.[30]

In Jung's view, when we pay attention to keeping open our attachments to the collective unconscious, to God, to models of the sublime, we move closer to power and wisdom and to going beyond the self.

Pain and trauma often give us the purpose to reconnect with our rhizome, our core being, our inner wholeness. As Beethoven suffered growing deafness, the sounds outside his head becoming fainter inside, his music grew in force and grandeur, raising the question of whether "he could have written that glorious paean of praise in the Ninth Symphony if he had not had to endure the dark closing in of deafness."[31] Milton was blind long before he undertook his epic. Writer Madeleine L'Engle wonders whether he could "have seen all that he sees in *Paradise Lost* if he had not been blind."[32] She also notes that "it is chastening to realize that those who have no physical flaw, who move through life in step with their peers, who are bright and beautiful, seldom become artists. The unending paradox is that we do learn through pain."[33]

SEARCHING OUT MEANING

There is no education like adversity.

—DISRAELI

Pain *is* a teacher, and purpose and meaning often emerge from what we learn. The "tremendous stress in a life-threatening illness" causes most everyone to "search out the meaning of their lives."[34] Rabbi Pesach Krauss, who served as chaplain at Memorial Sloan-Kettering Cancer Center in New York, says that people under such stress "often arrive at surprising answers (surprising because they are so obvious and so often overlooked) that apply to every human being—young, middle-aged, elderly—regardless of his or her health or station in life."[35]

One day Krauss asked a renowned scientist who was a patient at the hospital, "What has cancer taught you?" The scientist, who was facing death from his disease, had come a long way in his learning since he was admitted to the hospital some weeks before when he was depressed and angry about his condition. He said he had learned a number of things: first that he wasn't so "high and mighty" and that he'd better stop acting so arrogant "because I don't know it all." He also had learned that he was not in "complete control" of his life but that what he *could* control was his attitude. He had changed his attitude to be open to all experience, including the ordinary, and to be grateful. He told the rabbi:

> I've learned . . . that life is precious, that every moment has to count. I feel it when I get up in the morning and when I have a day without pain. It's amazing, it's like I'm reborn every day, capturing the wonder of another day. I feel as though there's an inner light shining. It's like—as you put it—the flow of God's mercy, or maybe nature's mercy, and it brings warmth like the sun's rays.[36]

This was coming from a man who had cut himself off from his wife, child, and colleagues in California because he had never placed much importance on relationships and the heart. Only the head counted. Now he was energized with new purpose, to take in, to consume, the joy and gift of being alive each day. Pointing to a red rose in a vase on the windowsill, he said:

> See that flower? I look at that rose like I've never seen a rose before. I'm sensitive to its color, the light and shadows playing on it, to its texture, and the way it's formed. What a marvelous, exquisite work of art, what a miracle it is . . . . [37]

This noted scientist had also discovered "how wonderful love is, too—the love of my child, the love of my wife. . . . I was always too busy to appreciate it. Now it's central and fresh, like that flower." He was going to leave the hospital soon and was committed to "triumphs in human relationships" in the time he had left, not just achievements in science. If this man had somehow experienced complete physical recovery, it would not have been as big a surprise—or miracle—as what he had found for himself as the meaning of his life.

Physical health is more of a means than an end. Many who have it and take it for granted are among those who keep seeking "something more." We need to be reminded that "health enables us to serve purpose in life, but it is not the purpose of life."[38] A friend of mine, Dr. Michael Hammond of Rice University, survived cancer to dedicate a beautiful new building for the Shepherd School of Music, where he serves as dean. He learned that "life is not about just feeling good but about being human and fully living. When one lives to the fullest, one suffers. The point is to suffer for a purpose."[39]

MALADIES THAT VANISHED

Age cannot wither her, nor custom stale

Her infinite variety.

—SHAKESPEARE

The purpose that opens space inside ourselves for other than pain is liberating. We are no longer slaves to a lust for more, we no longer follow the paths others insist we go on, we no longer fulfill the predictions doctors make about what we can and can't do or how long we have to live. One of my favorite Victorian women, Isabella Bird, was a liberated person in this sense. She had chronic back problems for much of her life, despite undergoing surgery at age 18 to remove a fibrous tumor from her spine and to relieve her pain.[40] When, depressed and depleted, she still had pain five years after the surgery, she left her sick bed and set out to travel. She sailed from Liverpool to visit a cousin in Canada and made a "startling" discovery[41]—her "maladies vanished" as long as she kept moving and challenging herself.[42] Whenever Bird returned home her pain, insomnia, and depression returned.

On her next trip, this time to Australia and New Zealand, she wrote her sister "at last I am in love."[43] Two days out of Auckland her ship was swept up in a South Sea hurricane. Suddenly, this "small, sick spinster from Edinburgh was aroused and tingling with life."[44] Although the storm raged for 12 hours and her steamer "nearly split asunder," Bird loved every minute of it.

Bird went from love of the sea to love of the mountains. She not only climbed the Rockies, becoming the first woman to scale the magnificent Long's Peak, but went from there to the top of the Himalayas and became a missionary in Tibet. Her purpose was literally as well as figuratively to keep climbing higher and reaching up to God.

What this amazing woman discovered is there are ways that strong purpose can keep us so committed and engaged that even pain cannot overtake the spirit. Pain may be, in fact, what leads us to the liberating experience where we make the discovery. After Bird's death in 1904 at age 73, the *Edinburgh Medical Journal* tried to explain the marvelous paradox that marked her life—"fragile, sensitive, and dependent," an "invalid" at home, yet a "Samson abroad" who "laughed at fatigue."[45] The journal editors could only conclude that she "was indeed one of those subjects who are dependent to the last degree upon their environment to bring out their possibilities" and to become so engaged that even pain is transcended.

Acute pain often carries a message that should not be ignored. It can tell us when something is wrong in the body and needs attention. For many of us, the hardest problem to deal with comes after the acute pain has received the best of attention and treatment and any tissue damage has been healed, but the pain hangs on in some form and becomes chronic—either as a persistent hurting, a gnawing ache, or a relentless sense of pressure. It is both the cause and effect of depression and despair. This is the kind of pain Bird came to realize she had and that only the discovery of something bigger in her life was going to liberate her from it.

SUPREME AND EXTREME GOALS

As soldiers, athletes, and performers know, purpose can transcend even acute pain. In remote areas of the world where initiation into manhood is a supreme goal of young males, painful rituals demonstrate how powerful such purpose is both psychologically and physically. In mountainous villages of parts of Central America, boys seeking to prove they are men are suspended from high wires by steel hooks inserted into their bare backs.[46] Dangling, they are transported by the network of wires from village to village, showing no evidence of pain. Similar hook-hanging rituals can be found in remote villages of India, where an honored young man is chosen to "channel the power of the gods into blessing the children and the harvest."[47] He travels from village to village, where he dangles from two swinging posts, with no sign of pain. After the ritual is over, observers report no evidence of infection or scar tissue from the hook-swinging.[48]

MAKING DEATH WAIT

People who make purpose part of their reason for being alive also make death wait. I remember Suzie, a 27-year-old woman who had multiple sclerosis and was dying of brain cancer at the inpatient unit where I began my hospice service. She was determined to live for her little boy's fifth birthday, which she did. On one of my visits with her, Suzie mentioned to me about how she had told her son to release a balloon on the day of her funeral and she would "catch it in heaven." I don't know if he did, but I believed Suzie when she said that because she loved country western music so much and used to dance the polka and Cotton Eyed Joe, she was going to dance up a storm in heaven.

I also won't forget the wife of a longtime colleague, Dr. Richard Shekelle. Sue, a 51-year-old geriatric social worker at Baylor College of Medicine, was so determined to live life to the fullest that by the time she died of cancer she had climbed the Himalayas in Nepal, run a half-marathon, and skydived twice. She also steeped herself in the beauty of Pacific sunsets and the art of the masters. Rick and Sue had moved from Houston to Southern California after her cancer metastasized to her lungs. Only four months before her death, while she was still recovering from surgery and radiation on her mouth and oral cavity, the primary site of her cancer, a nephew offered her a once-in-a-lifetime invitation to attend a special preview in New York of paintings of Picasso that had never been exhibited before. She excitedly bought a black evening gown and elbow-length black gloves and pumps and boarded a plane in Los Angeles. In New York, a picture was taken of her in her elegant evening attire, which was used on the back page of her memorial program four months later. After the preview at the Museum of Modern Art and a formal dinner, she returned to her hotel at 2 AM, then boarded a plane the next day back to Los Angeles, where her husband picked her up. The same spring, she made her skydiving debut and liked it so well she went back for a second dive. She died in July 1996; at her memorial in Houston, my wife, Rita, remarked to Rick, "She made sure her gas tank was empty when she died." Sue used determination to make death wait until it was empty.

LIVING FOR PASSOVER

Elisabeth Kübler-Ross was one of the first to report the observation that dying patients often enter a "bargaining phase" in which they ask God to allow them to live until an important occasion, which may be the wedding of a son or daughter or grandchild, the birth of a grandchild, a birthday, an anniversary, Christmas, or Easter.[49] Whether they perceive God as the source of the strength to survive or not, such patients possess a purpose that gives profound meaning to their remaining life.

To test this hypothesis scientifically, sociologists David P. Phillips and Elliot W. King of the University of California at San Diego examined death certificates across 18 years of 1,919 Jewish people in California. In a paper in the British medical journal, *The Lancet,* entitled "Death Takes a Holiday: Mortality Surrounding Major Social Occasions,"[50] the researchers reported that "the number of deaths was lower than expected in the week before Passover and higher than expected in the week after."[51] The death dip and peak did not occur among various control groups, including African-Americans, Asian-Americans, and Jewish infants. The authors concluded that the Passover has such importance to Jewish adults that it is associated with the prolonging of life. The Passover effect, they added, may be "just one in a general category of patterns associated with important, religious, political, and social occasions."[52]

Birthdays may also give resolve and purpose to those who are dying. For example, both Thomas Jefferson and John Adams died on July 4, 1826, 50 years after the birthday of the Declaration of Independence. Jefferson's physician was at his bedside when the former president asked in a husky, indistinct voice, "Is it the Fourth?" The doctor replied, "It soon will be."[53] Jefferson, founding father of the Declaration, waited until the fourth to die.

LIVING TO PAINT AND PLEASE

Why stay on the earth except to grow?

—ROBERT BROWNING

The desire to carry out the wishes of someone we feel very close to or highly respect can also have a prolonging effect on life. Dr.

Don Carlos Peete of Kansas City, beloved by patients and fellow physicians alike across more than a half century of medical practice, told of an engraver whose wife had died a few years earlier at age 80.[54] Peete had cared for both for many years. When the husband was hospitalized for signs of heart failure, he told the doctor that he had had a good life and had finished his "accomplishments," so Peete "shouldn't take too much trouble" in keeping him alive.

The doctor then remembered the lovely paintings the engraver had hanging in his apartment, all his own work. Peete told him: "You must get well and paint me a picture." The patient perked up immediately and replied: "If that's what you want, I will do it for you."

> It was surprising how quickly he got well. Soon he was down in Penn Valley Park on a bright summer's day painting a picture for me. He lived five more years to almost 90 years of age. We have the painting as one of our prizes.

Many years earlier, when Peete himself was 5 years old, he had been stricken with lobar pneumonia and was in a coma for a time. "Our doctor was a big, tall man with a beard and drove a horse and buggy. I remember it was an extremely cold winter day and he wore a heavy fur coat. He was very kind and gentle and after listening to my chest, taking my temperature and pulse, he patted me on the cheek and said: 'You are going to get well.'" Peete not only hoped he would, he was determined. He didn't want to let his doctor down. It was his first lesson in how powerful the effect of a good doctor can be.

DYING TO MUSIC

As the sun colors flowers, so does art color life.
—SIR JOHN LUBBOCK

How well we die (see Chapter 10) may be more important than when. Families of the dying often bring treasured photographs and music to the bedside of their loved one at hospice in hopes death will be made easier. I want to die hearing the andante of Mozart's Piano Concerto 21, Beethoven's Ninth Symphony's *Ode to Joy,* a Puccini aria, and just about anything by Bach, whether it is a concerto, fugue, suite, or oratorio. I like Bach and Beethoven for different reasons, as explained by this comparison:

> Bach's music is transcendent, but Beethoven's music
> is about our struggle to transcend.
> Unlike Bach, he could rage.
> Through his deafness he discovered an aspect of chaos.
> His music beats chaos down.
> Order triumphs, at least in art.[55]

I believe that when beauty has been a passion and purpose in our lives, it may serve an even bigger purpose in our dying. There is evidence that although dying patients may be in a coma, they still respond to voices and music and to the touch of those they love.

When Leonard Bernstein went for the last time to visit Nadia Boulanger, his old counterpoint teacher who had deep influence on musicians and conductors of the 20th Century in both this country and Europe, he was told she would not recognize him, she was in a coma and dying. "I was ushered into her bedchamber," Bernstein said, "by the angelic and anxiety-ridden Mademoiselle

Dieudonne, who, with forefinger to lips, and seconded by an attending nurse, whispered a sharp order: ten minutes only...."[56]

Despite being almost totally blind and infirm, Boulanger had stayed active with her music, teaching and talking, until she was 90. "....she had uncomplainingly surrendered more of her body to the earth, so there must have seemed very little left for death to claim, but her spirit remained indomitable."[57] Bernstein knelt "in silent communion" by the bed of his mentor, now 92. Suddenly, he heard her voice, as strong as ever:

"Who is there?"

Bernstein answered, "Lenny, Leonard...." Then there was silence again. "Cher Lenny..." Bernstein thought, she *knew;* a "miracle." He asked her how she felt. After a pause, Mademoiselle Boulanger replied: "Quite strong."

"You mean...inside yourself?" Bernstein asked.

"Yes. But the flesh—." He said he understood, that she must be very tired. She replied, "No tiredness. None." He got up to go, but the voice commanded, "Don't leave."

He heard himself asking, "Do you hear music in your head?" She replied instantly, "All the time." What was she hearing now, he inquired. Bernstein remembered her loves were Mozart, Monteverdi, Bach, Stravinsky, and Ravel.

There was a long pause. "One music," she said, "with no beginning, no end." He felt that "she was already there, on the other side."[58] She had merged into the music that had been the passion and purpose of her life. And she was well inside herself.

Chapter Eight

FINDING

FAITH

Faith is the force of life.

—TOLSTOY

The question we have been dealing with in this book is how people gain and retain a sense of health or well-being when they are sick and hurting. Since the evidence suggests that well-being can exist side by side with pain and illness, we have been exploring ways by which we access this deeper level of health. Faith is one of the ways.

Faith, as well as pain, purpose, and appreciation, can lead us to a sense of being whole because it helps us connect to larger identities. So what is faith and where does it come from? "Some people distinguish between *belief* (by which they mean ideas they hold to be true), *trust* (the confidence they feel in someone else), and *faith* (believing where we cannot prove)," observes one scholar on the subject.[1] If we look to the Bible, where these words often appear, there are no such distinctions among them in both the Hebrew of the Torah and the Greek of the New Testament.[2] Faith, then, is a feeling, a conviction, a knowing that is both cognitive and affective, coming from both head and heart. To me, it isn't blind acceptance or an ignoring of facts. The facts are that pain as well as joy comes with life, that bad things happen to good people, and that value can be found in the bad as well as the good. Faith does not come from being guaranteed that there is a God or divine creator. My conception of God is of an ineffable being infinitely greater than anything the mortal mind can fathom, so human "proof" of

God's existence is not within our grasp. Blaise Pascal, the 17th Century genius who was both an inventor and mathematician as well as a philosopher, offered this proposition to those whose faith requires guarantees: Act as if there is a God. Even if there isn't, you will still benefit by acting as though there were. If there is a God, you will be at least two times better off. What do you have to lose?[3]

The facts are that faith gives strength, solace, and perseverance to millions of people, particularly those with pain and disease as constant companions. For many, it inspires and motivates. For all, it offers a cognitive and emotional map to guide us through turmoil and trouble.[4] In so doing, it provides us with the coherence that is a cornerstone to a sense of well-being and health.

THE WAY THE BRAIN IS BUILT

Faith is . . . the conviction of things not seen.

—HEBREWS

The great philosopher genius, Immanuel Kant, who is ranked in importance with Plato and Aristotle, understood that the stirrings of the human heart toward "higher truths"—God, immortality, justice, freedom—can quicken the soul and instill in us a passion for life. God's existence, Kant argued, cannot be proved, because rational, empirical proof belongs to the observable while God is "noumenal" (intuited) and transcendent.[5]

Dr. Herbert Benson of Harvard has suggested that humans are "wired for God," that throughout the history of the species, people have demonstrated faith in "something beyond" and that religious belief is "second nature" to us.[6] If we look at such belief for its survival value, there is no denying that faith helps people to survive, and the evidence is clear that religious and spiritual commitment is strongly correlated not only with health but happiness.[7]

The capacity to transcend, to have coherence, faith, and an experience of God is "a consequence of the brain's construction,"[8] which in turn is guided by something deeper. Neuropsychologist Michael Persinger notes that all of us have the capacity to experience God.

> Some of us may regress to it, others may enhance it, still others may be embarrassed by its presence. Like the propensity to walk, to talk, it is a potential in each of us. We may just know it by different names.[9]

Both writers and scientists have studied the propensity, calling it by various names. William Faulkner believed that "man in his essence" will slowly keep improving a little, because the core impulse to reach higher, to be better, is an insistent one, a restless urge that will not leave us alone.[10] This innate urge to go beyond the self are what the Columbia University historians referred to as the needs of the human spirit and the call to transcendence (see Chapter 2). Geneticist Theodosius Dobyzhansky identified the core impulse as the urgent, indispensable element in us that gives our lives depth and our spirit ultimate meaning.[11] Anthropologist Ashley Montagu insists it is the "vitalizing drive" that makes us complete as human beings.[12] Rousseau simply called it our "religious impulse,"[13] *religio* or *religare* standing for that innermost part that ties us to something bigger.

Dr. Eric Cassell, in the *New England Journal of Medicine,* said the evidence is universal that humans have a "transcendent dimension," which enlivens us and fuels our spirit.[14] Though largely ignored by the medical profession, it is found not only in religion but in "intense feelings" of bonding with other people, groups, ideas, nature, art, music, and it can bestow a sense of inner health and belonging to something bigger and more enduring than a single life.

TUNING IN TO SOMETHING LARGER

I knew an atheist novelist who used to say prayers every night . . . 80 percent of our writers, if only they could avoid putting their names to it, would write and hail the name of God.

—CAMUS

Sir Alexander Hardy, the biologist and fellow of the Royal Society who founded the Religious Experience Research Unit at Oxford after becoming convinced that such experience is "widespread" though neglected by science, agreed that "it takes more than a sophisticated sneer to dismiss it all as illusion."[15] The first Soviet cosmonaut came back from space reporting, if not with a sneer, then with confirmed disbelief, that he had just travelled the heavens and no God was there. In contrast, Edgar Mitchell, on the Apollo 14 mission, returned with a strong faith in transcendence:

> There was a vast tranquility, a growing sense of wonder as I looked out the window. . . . Somehow I felt tuned into something much larger than myself, something much larger than the planet in the window. . . . there was . . . a feeling of ubiquitous harmony—a sense of interconnectedness. . . I experienced what has been described as an ecstasy of unity. I not only *saw* the connectedness, I *felt* it and experienced it sentiently.[16]

What the wounded but well have done is to make full use of their faith in the transcendent, to feel part of something larger. They have found wholeness beyond the physical body by emphasizing the nonphysical self.[17] The physical self seeks material ease, comfort, and pleasure, and many of us in the West are privileged to enjoy a high standard of living by objective measures. However, as theologian and religion scholar Huston Smith reminds us, the physical self "cannot satisfy the human heart completely" no matter how much affluence or success it achieves materially. Even if we accumulate all the wealth or power or success or bodily health we ever hoped for, the physical and material dimension will not give everyday life the vitality, richness, and joy we yearn for.

As we saw in the last chapter, acquiring material things is a means, not an end. Both scientists and nonscientists alike have concluded that we possess an innate urge, impulse, and capacity for a "more" that the world of material experience cannot requite. Like trees and plants that keep reaching and bending for the light that nourishes them, we keep looking up for more, and when we connect with something higher, deeper, or finer, we are inspirited, as if new breath has infused us—which it has.

Because we are, then, "wired for God" and have the capacity for transcendence, taking Pascal up on his proposition should not be that hard, even when we begin with deep doubt and disbelief. But, as Pascal intuited, for the biology of belief to be activated, the neural pathways by which faith is experienced require us to expose ourselves to God, and if we must, to "act as if" we believe.

Practicing Before Believing

Practicing faith is a common doorway to belief. The most powerful way humans come to believe something is by observing and imitating the behavior of those around them who model that behavior. When I began mountain climbing, I practiced the behavior of friends who were veterans at doing it. I had faith in them. My faith preceded my belief that I could do mountains.

I began a practice of daily prayers before I believed it would do any good. I began when I was so depressed that there wasn't much else to do. Prozac wasn't working and in fact was making me nauseated and more anxious and agitated. Another antidepressant, Pamelor, relieved my fearful middle-of-the night ruminations. But I still felt at a distance from people and my work during the day. I resolved to act as if I had faith in God and began the practice of daily prayers, morning and afternoon. Slowly, the reexperiencing of genuine faith came, followed by belief. The same sequence occurred when I started attending Twelve-Step programs for those with family members and loved ones addicted to alcohol and drugs. Alcoholics Anonymous, the first of these programs, is clear about "fake it to make it," meaning participate, act like the recovered alcoholics, and keep working the program even if at first it feels strange, artificial, or mechanical.

In the Colorado Rockies, I have had the experience on climbs of having faith that I would reach the top of a mountain but not believing I could. One year after Rita and I took our daughter's ashes to distribute at Blue Lake high in the Indian Peaks, I wanted to return, but I had chronic swelling and pain in my right knee from an injury in two falls in the mountains during the past summer. I truly doubted I could climb the three miles up to the lake, but faith that I would sustained me and lifted me above my pain. My knee even felt better after the climb than it did before. Because faith is larger than belief, it can accommodate doubts, skepticism, even agnosticism, any of which is bound to occur at one time or another when pain persists.

FAITH AND DISBELIEF

There lives more faith in honest doubt,
Believe me, than in half the creeds.

—TENNYSON

My experience is that many of us believe, but we need help with
our "unbelief."[18] For me, practicing faith despite disbelief is akin to
"grabbing aholt of God" and not letting go until we are blessed.
That phrase came from Walker Percy, a physician who got tuberculosis while performing autopsies at Bellevue Hospital and transformed his illness into a career as a best-selling novelist. Percy died
of cancer in 1990 but had already decided that "I don't see why
anyone should settle for anything less than Jacob, who actually
grabbed aholt of God and wouldn't let go until God identified
himself and blessed him."[19]

Genesis depicts Jacob as wrestling with the Angel of God, suffering a laming injury in the struggle but getting his blessing,
which stayed with him the rest of his long life. I like to think that
all the wounded but well will be specially blessed, like Jacob, if we
just grab hold of what faith stands for and persist despite struggle
and pain.

Because our pain and "wounds" can get us down, we may become so weary and low that we lose our hold. Bishop Geralyn
Wolf (Chapter 4) says that during her recuperation from breast
cancer surgery and chemotherapy, "she was so tired, confused or
anxious" at times that she wondered what had become of her faith.
She felt like the apostles who fell asleep at Gethsemane when Jesus
asked them to watch over him as he prayed. But, as she thought
about it, "I can see that, even when I fell asleep, that Jesus did not
sleep. That he was praying in me."[20]

SPIRITUAL IMMERSION OF A SCIENTIST

In my most extreme fluctuations, I have never been an atheist in the sense of denying the existence of God.

—DARWIN

The English biologist and author Rupert Sheldrake (Chapter 4) tells of "outgrowing" any belief or faith in God after his scientific education at Cambridge. "I had a typical secular-humanist atheistic worldview for a long time, well into my thirties."[21] Then in 1968 he went to India and "all the materialist assumptions I took for granted just didn't seem to work anymore." What he found was a culture where the idea of "other realms"—the supernatural or spiritual—"was simply taken for granted by practically everybody. There was a palpable sense of another dimension to life, everywhere you looked, and everywhere you went."

Sheldrake's initial reaction as an atheist was to think that all these people were deluded. But the fact he could not deny was that the culture of spiritual beliefs worked. "Even people living in the extremes of poverty seemed to have more joy in their lives than most people I knew who lived in the lap of plenty. I was touched deeply by the natural human warmth, and the quality of the people and of their way of life." Sheldrake had been brought up on the idea that materialism, not spirituality, made people happy.

> The people there were poor beyond the comprehension of most Westerners, yet everywhere they walked about with the most radiant smiles. Walk along a street in London, Paris or New York and you see mostly harried, worried faces. That difference impressed me very deeply.[22]

The contrast Sheldrake experienced between "the sense of inner joy and peace" all around him in India compared with "the tense way of life in the West" was so striking that he decided to take up various forms of Hindu practice, starting with meditation. From it, "I experienced within myself that calm I was seeing all around me in India."[23]

A Return to Roots

Teach me, O God, not to torture myself, not to make a martyr of myself through stifling reflection, but rather teach me to breathe deeply in faith.

—KIERKEGAARD

After following Hindu practices for four years while living and working in India as a scientist, Sheldrake came to realize that "there was no way I'd ever be an Indian. I began to have a sense that I would need to recover my own tradition if I were to share in the deep perceptions and peace that I saw in the people around me."[24]

Sheldrake abandoned atheism and returned to his Christian heritage, which he found more optimistic than what he believed was the case with the fatalism of Hindu belief. Gradually he gave up meditation for prayer. "I would say that meditation involves a kind of separation between the practice and the rest of one's life; it is going into another space altogether." With petitionary and intercessory prayer, he found a way to link the events of daily life with spiritual practice.

> I pray about what I've done that day and what's coming up the next day. It's a matter of bringing the very fabric of one's life—relationships, work, and personal concerns—into the context of the spiritual life.[25]

Faith, then, comes to us from different directions, but whatever path is used, practice—through rituals, worship, prayer, or the kind of immersion in a spiritual environment that Sheldrake had—is necessary to spark the neuronal pathways that make the experience of God a conscious, physical reality. Once the experience occurs, God becomes a felt presence. The facts of faith are that not only is it good for us, it is an essential mainstay for those who live with chronic or recurring disease or disability and have to deal frequently with pain or trauma.

DELORES' SENSE OF A PRESENCE

Delores, 38, a participant in our breast cancer study who later developed metastases to the neck and shoulders, lives with the faith that God is present in her daily life.[26] She felt that presence guiding her before she was first diagnosed in May 1992. She had quit her job after seven years as a newspaper carrier. "I had gotten my affairs straightened out and things fell into place just before I was diagnosed." Although she was a single parent with three young children, had no savings and no insurance, she managed to get a mammogram two days after she felt a lump in her breast and was admitted to the hospital in a week and a half. "After surgery, which I thought was going to be the only treatment I needed, they wanted to start me on chemotherapy. I said I would have to think it over." Over the next several days she prayed hard for guidance. "I got up one morning and felt like someone was pouring warm pudding over my head. I felt the distinct presence of God and a peace came over me. I knew, then, I was being guided to go ahead with the chemo, and everything would be all right." She felt annointed.

The round of drugs left Delores without hair but never made her sick or produced other side-effects. Her explanation is that "I was at peace with the chemo. I was willing to do it; it wasn't a forced thing." More than two years later, she started having pains in her shoulder and couldn't raise one arm. She had an MRI, which detected a hole in her scapula from metastatic cancer. "I had just been diagnosed again with cancer and I found myself singing in the car on the way home. Suddenly I wasn't upset anymore. I was calm and peaceful and sensed God's presence."

Later, cancer was found in her cervical spine, and she was put in a neck brace, which she wore 24 hours a day for months. "I made up my mind I wasn't going to live in a neck brace, and I gradually stopped wearing it." The piece of broken bone in her neck surprisingly "reattached."

Delores has lost her hair twice from two rounds of chemotherapy. "I look for the positive in every experience. I tell people losing my hair has advantages. I don't have to shampoo it. I don't have to pay money for hair cuts." Each time her hair has grown back it has turned darker and changed texture. "It's now just the way I have always wanted it. It is black and curly. It used to be brown, almost blond, and straight."

In the midst of her cancer and its recurrence, Delores has had to deal with other crises. Her husband left her, began drinking heavily again, lost his job and truck, and now lives in a homeless shelter. She and her children moved in with her mother and live on Delores' disability pay, which is less than half the income she used to have.

Delores leads a Bible class at her church and works with others in a support group for cancer patients. She has made prayer a daily routine. "I don't pray at any set time; I pray all day long to myself and don't say "amen" until the end of the day." She says she believes she can "feel comfortable with any situation, no matter how bad."

She doesn't think about dying. "The doctors say I will die with the bone cancer but not from it. I think God has a plan for my life, and I won't die soon. When I do, I won't fear death."

EVIDENCE OF PRAYER'S EFFECTIVENESS

Prayer is the slender nerve that moves the muscle of Omnipotence.

—J. E. HARTILL

Dossey, who has written a number of fine books on spirituality, medicine, and health, recalls that as a young physician he had "a patient with metastatic lung cancer who was dying."[27] The patient refused all medical and surgical interventions and used prayer as "therapy." Members of his church prayed for him "around the clock." Dossey "sent him home to die." A year later, a colleague at Dossey's hospital phoned him to say, "You ought to see your old patient. He's back in the hospital with a bad case of flu." Dossey was "stunned. I dashed to the radiology department for a look at his latest chest x-ray." There was no sign of cancer. The report of the radiologist, who assumed the patient had been given chemotherapy, said: "In the intervening twelve months there has been a dramatic response to therapy." The radiologist didn't know that the patient's only treatment was prayer.

Perplexed, Dossey sought an explanation from two medical school professors. One said: "Don't be troubled. We see this." The other responded, "This is simply the 'natural course' of this disease." The "explanations" didn't help the young doctor, but "I did what most doctors do when confronted with these inexplicable phenomena: I ignored it. It took me many years to gather enough courage to confront these events without cringing."[28]

Scientific medicine cannot accept prayer as having any effect because prayer implies "action at a distance," and there is no scientific law to explain such a phenomenon. In the 1600s Kepler ran into the same problem when he proposed that the Earth's tides were "caused by the tug of lunar gravity."[29] Outraged, "Galileo, the most prestigious scientist of the day, declared, 'These are the ravings of a madman! Kepler believes in action at a distance!'" Marconi, the inventor of radio, received similar treatment when he "proposed that invisible waves could circulate through space and carry intelligible information at enormous distances." He was considered crazy and temporarily committed to an insane asylum.[30]

After a number of years of ignoring clinical examples of patients being benefited by prayer, Dossey began searching out reports in the world literature documenting the effects. He was so impressed by the experimental evidence that he found on prayer that he resolved to start using prayer in his medical practice.[31] The experimental evidence includes research of the Spendrift research group in Pennsylvania that has measured the effects of prayer on plants and other organisms, which allow tightly controlled studies. Controlled research is necessary to rule out other possible causes of the effects observed. Because of the rigorous methodology employed, "the positive results are not easily attributable to suggestion, expectation, or positive thinking—the so-called placebo effect."[32]

Dossey also came across 131 controlled trials reported by Daniel J. Benor, M.D., in Germany, showing statistically significant effects of prayer on enzymes, cells, yeasts, bacteria, plants, animals, and human beings.[33] Convinced by these studies and others, Dossey began using a nondirected prayer for his patients, along the lines of, "May the best outcome occur for this patient," and "May thy will be done."[34]

SHOULD PHYSICIANS PRESCRIBE PRAYER?

With the growing evidence on prayer, well-being, and health, the *Journal of the American Medical Association (JAMA)* has asked in an article on the subject: "Should physicians write 'prayer' or 'more frequent participation in religious observances' when prescribing for their patients?"[35] Prayer, faith in God, and Bible reading—"typical types of Judeo-Christian behavior"—have been found to be effective in preventing depression in the presence of severe disabilities, such as serious heart disease and diabetes. In one study, the most disabled persons showed the highest religious coping and the lowest depression. The researcher reported that "it did not necessarily prevent the disability, but it did prevent or reduce the depression that accompanies disability."[36]

Controlled studies outside the United States have shown similar results. In a 16-year prospective study of 11 religious and 11 matched secular kibbutzim in Israel, belonging to a religious collective was associated with a strong protective effect against the risk of death.[37] Mortality was considerably higher in the secular kibbutzim, controlling for confounding factors such as sociodemographic variables. The paper, appearing in the *American Journal of Public Health,* asked: "Does religious observance promote health?" The answer was yes.

A stronger immune system may be one physical benefit people receive from regular attendance at religious services, suggesting that both spiritual community and practice of prayer are helpful. Recent evidence from epidemiological studies at Duke University Medical Center shows that among 1,718 persons age 65 and above, those who attended services at least once a week had "healthier" immune function as measured by Interleukin-6 markers, than did non-attenders.[38]

Another study in Israel has looked at the effects of "healing intention operating at a distance" on hospitalized patients undergoing herniotomy (surgical repair of a hernia). Researchers found a positive, "significant difference in those receiving healing intention" from distant sites without the patients' knowledge. They recovered faster from surgery and had fewer complications than those in a control group and a third group who received only suggestion."[39]

As to the faith of physicians and scientists and their beliefs about God, two recent surveys have reported surprising results. In a 1997 survey of leading U.S. scientists (physicists, biologists, and mathematicians), about 40 percent said they believed in a personal God to whom one may pray "in expectation of receiving an answer."[40] Using the same questions as a 1916 survey, a questionnaire was sent in 1996 to 1,000 randomly selected scientists and got close to the same results as the survey 80 years earlier. Despite a great rise in secular attitudes and skepticism since 1916 and despite more questions raised as to God's existence, the percent of believing scientists remained stable.

As to physicians, who have professed more belief when questioned than scientists, a 1996 study by the American Academy of Family Physicians showed that 99 percent of doctors "believe an important relationship exists between the spirit and the flesh and many see prayer as a means of helping heal the sick.[41]

PRAYER NETWORKS

Deidre Henneman, a nurse convinced of the efficacy of prayer, organized a whole network of strangers to pray for her when she underwent stem cell replacement and high doses of chemotherapy to treat her metastasized cancer in the liver and lung.[42] She had undergone a double mastectomy for breast cancer in May 1994 and reconstruction surgery in February 1995 when the metastasis was diagnosed.

After writing her will and making funeral arrangements in case she never came home, Henneman entered the Midwestern Regional Medical Center in Zion, Illinois, where she would be in total isolation for a month after the stem cell replacement, a procedure similar to bone marrow transplant. She knew no one in that part of the country, so before she was hospitalized, she called churches in Zion and asked if they could send people to visit her during her isolation. With the help of three churches, she had a visitor every day.

> We talked and prayed together. One day, I couldn't do even that, so my visitor just read to me. That was wonderful. . . . Another woman played the flute. I knew these encouraging visits were the answers to my prayers.

Henneman also arranged for her friends and family around the country to pray for her. "On some days," she said, "I'm sure I had 2,000 people praying for me, including 1,000 people in Zion alone."[43] Henneman was in remission by April 1996, when she was found free of tumors in the lung and liver.

Churches throughout the nation have prayer teams and networks not only to pray for those in special need but to offer prayers each day for their members, sick or well, with or without their knowledge. At one church I know of with a prayer network, the name of a member came up to be prayed for at the 5:30 PM services. This was the very time he was driving home from a business meeting outside of Houston and was involved in a serious collision, which sent him and his car hurtling into the bank of a deep ditch. His car was demolished, but he escaped with only scrapes and bruises. His rector said, "Bob was surrounded by those prayers" and protected by them.

Prayer has the power to act at a distance, Dossey believes, which means it is not some form of energy, which physics tells us weakens as distance increases. Whatever it is, many patients like Deidre Henneman who experience remission and healing of life-threatening disease or those who may miraculously escape serious injury are convinced that prayer is largely responsible.

A PEAK EXPERIENCE

We walk by faith, not by sight.

—*II CORINTHIANS*

A time of physical danger as well as life-threatening illness elicits repeated prayers of entreaty from most all of us when we find ourselves in such circumstances. Rita and I were trapped by bad weather atop Long's Peak, one of America's most challenging and highest climbs. Low clouds and fog rolled in, making it impossible to find our way off of the 14,255-foot mountain. The guidance system for climbers at the summit and the long rocky stretch of ledges back to what is called the Keyhole consists of red and yellow bullseyes painted at varying distances by rangers on the side of slabs of granite and boulders. On the August afternoon when we began our descent, we couldn't spot the bullseyes because of the fog and clouds. Others ahead of us had scrambled down before the bad weather set in. So we were on our own.

I began praying in earnest. If we didn't keep going down, nightfall would overtake us before we could reach the Keyhole and the Boulderfield beyond, where we could fashion shelter for the night. But to try to keep moving without guidance was equally hazardous because of the precipitous drop-offs from the ledges we had to traverse. Our prayers for clearing weather and a safe descent were not answered immediately or as we had hoped. But we discovered that if we kept peering ahead to where we guessed the next bullseye should be, the fog would slowly lift just long enough for us to get a glimpse of red and yellow. The glimpse was enough to give us direction for our next 30-40 yards or so. After this pattern kept occurring, I started praying for the glimpse of just one bullseye at a time rather than for the sight of the sun breaking through the fog and clouds. We crawled and scrambled from one red and yellow circle to another and after what seemed like a lifetime, we made it before dark through the Keyhole formation into the massive Boulderfield below, still many hours from the trailhead but largely out of danger.

Recounting and reliving the experience as we continued our descent, we both agreed we had had a religious experience. I had recently reread William James' *The Varieties of Religious Experience* but couldn't recall one like ours. In any case, we both felt we had been given unforgettable evidence of the power of prayer. Our "incredible journey," as Rita described it on the climbers' register at the rangers station when we returned in moonlight, took 18 hours 20 minutes.

ANGER AT GOD BY THE STRICKEN

But the age-old question is, why do some prayers get results and others don't? A person in pain or threat of dying whose prayers go unanswered is often just as deserving as the one whose prayers are answered. Theologians have wrestled for centuries with the problem of theodicy and the question of how a loving God can allow the innocent to suffer. The classic "case study" from the Bible is, of course, Job. He was a generous, godly man blessed with everything until disease, death, and destruction wiped out his family, fortune, and health, leaving him sitting in pain and ashes on a dung heap, protesting his innocence and demanding that God answer why all this tragedy was heaped on him. Job never received an explanation, but he got something more powerful and lasting. God appears to him out of a whirlwind and Job is face to face with his living God. Job is humbled and satisfied. "I had heard of thee by the hearing of the ear, but now my eye sees thee...," Job confesses. Having the experience of the presence of God and the knowledge that "my redeemer liveth" was more than enough for Job. Some of the women I interviewed in the breast cancer study wanted an explanation from God, at first, for why they were being faced with a life-threatening crisis. As I mentioned, a few not only demanded an answer but also wanted God to know how angry they were. Most, however, didn't ever raise the "Why me?" question, which is a finding also reported by other researchers studying people struck by various calamities.[44] For these women, their faith remained steadfast. Some felt called to show that something of value can come from any disaster; others felt confident that God would reveal what plan he had for them as time went on.

FAITH THAT THERE IS A PLAN

Jacquelyn, who had a modified radical mastectomy and chemotherapy, is one who has faith that there is a plan for her, although she doesn't know what it is.[45] She uses prayer daily to deal not only with the experience of having had cancer but all else she has to handle in her busy life as a manager in a large corporation and the mother of three children, two of whom are teenagers. At 40, she is the "fixer" and problem-solver in her family, and her faith, she says, helps her feel less alone. Jacquelyn's faith has been with her since she was a child, and she is convinced she will always have it.

Lilly (see Chapters 3 and 6) moved even closer to God and strengthened her faith as her breast cancer became stage IV and metastasized to the spine. She believes quality of life can be measured in both spiritual and physical terms. Physically, she now has trouble doing even simple household chores, but she now identifies "more with the spiritual part" of herself and says that she "feels better emotionally" and is "more at peace with herself and God and her life than ever before."[46] Lilly would agree, as Peter Gomes of Harvard (Chapter 4) puts it: "Death is real. The body is real" but "the spirit is also real, in fact, more real than death or the body, each of which, when it has done its work, disappears."[47] To enhance the spirit, we must remind ourselves that "we are not simply material people in a material world"; we are more than "prisoners of the flesh."[48]

An Inner, Felt Knowledge

Knowledge, like religion, must be "experienced" in order to be known.

—HENRY WHIPPLE

Jacquelyn, Lilly, and the majority of the other women in the cancer study cannot articulate why they believe in God or have faith. They just "know" they do. The integrative biologist Michael Polanyi[49] identified two kinds of knowing—explicit knowledge and tacit knowledge. The explicit can be expressed in words, mathematical symbols, diagrams, and maps. The tacit comes in the act of experiencing, of responding, of doing and being. Sir Arthur Conan Doyle, the English physician who became famous as the creator of Sherlock Holmes, in affirming his spiritual faith, said: "It is not that I think or that I believe . . . but that I know."[50]

So when we experience the presence of God, we have inner knowledge on which faith stands. It is the "evidence" that the unknown author of the *Epistle to the Hebrews* referred to when he said "faith is . . . the evidence of things not seen."[51] Job had the exceptional experience of seeing his God, but he already had inner knowledge of God's existence, for his faith never wavered throughout his trials and tribulations.

MASSIVE INHUMANITY AND FAITH

But, for others, tragedy can destroy faith or be used to "prove" faith is foolish. A calamity can be so mammoth, such as the Holocaust, that anger at God will never leave for some, and others have died, or will die, convinced there is no God for allowing such massive inhumanity. I felt physically ill, and Rita actually got sick for days, after we visited Bergen-Belsen, the prisoner camp of the Nazis where Anne Frank died just a few weeks before the British Army liberated the remaining survivors in April 1945. Anne Frank was a truly remarkable young woman, as her diary demonstrates, but she had to have strong faith to give her the joy of life and the hunger for beauty that sustained her right up to the time the Nazis carted her and her family away to imprisonment and death.

For those who lose faith from the inhumanity of a Bergen-Belsen, there is an event that happened on the day the camp was liberated that has stayed with me to enlarge my faith. The means of execution at Belsen was not the gas chamber or the gallows but starvation. The British moved trucks in loaded with bread. They were feeding the starved survivors starting at the far reaches of the camp first. Not far from the entrance, though, a truck made a turn too sharply and two loaves of bread fell to the ground. A knot of emaciated, bedraggled, half-dead men, women, and children circled around the food and, for what two British correspondents said seemed like a lifetime, nothing happened. No one spoke. No one dived for the bread. No one pushed the women and children out of the way. Finally, in an exquisite violation of Darwinian law, two of the male ex-prisoners quietly picked up the loaves, broke them into equal pieces, and began feeding the women and children.

Frankl (Chapter 3), a resilient survivor of Auschwitz and Dachau, came out convinced that meaning and purpose in life saved him and will keep anyone alive, regardless of the hardship, if held onto.[52] Many people, including those in our study, use their religion and faith in God to give their lives meaning.

Meaning is so powerful because it helps answer the gnawing, fundamental question of *why*. Why are we here at all, much less why must we have pain? The philosopher Nietzsche said that humans can bear any *what* if they know the *why*. Healing itself relates to why we are around, to our purpose in existing. It is not enough, psychiatrist Gerald May observes, to discover *how* to overcome depression or to be cured of a disease or disorder.[53] We want to know *why*—why live at all?

Spirituality measures that researchers have developed to study whether meaning is associated with health and well-being apply to both people who participate in an organized religion and those who perceive themselves as spiritual outside of religion. The evidence suggests that spirituality, both within religion and external to it, is associated with well-being.[54] A large longitudinal study tracking the health of thousands of adults in Kauai, the San Francisco Bay Area and Arizona indicates that spirituality is a powerful predictor of vitality in aging.[55] Meaning and purpose are seen as central to measures of spirituality.

BOTH PEACE AND JOY

May the road rise up to meet you.

May the wind be always at your back.

May the sun shine warm upon your face.

And the rains fall soft upon your fields. . . .

—AN IRISH BLESSING

After observing an equanimity and peace in so many of the women with cancer who have strong faith, and after listening to them about God having a plan for their lives, I could see that they knew why they were here. Judeo-Christian beliefs hold that we're here to love God, to tend the garden or vineyard—the world we have been given—and to love one another, which are themes reflected in other major religions.[56] Peace comes from knowing we are doing these things the best we can. We have faith that we are fulfilling the charge we have been given and that brings peace even in the midst of pain.

But there is more. There is also joy. The women I have met and spent time with have a surprising joy, even those who have suffered recurrences of their cancer and live with physical pain. Perhaps I should say particularly those who now are in or are moving toward the advanced stages of cancer, because I would include Delores and Lilly among these who have an inspiring joy. Dr. Roy Mathew, a physician on the faculty of Duke University Medical Center, comes closest to explaining the very biological basis of this joy.[57]

From PET scans and other brain studies, he has concluded that dopamine—our primary "pleasure" neurochemical—is most consistently activated and sustained when we make larger connections in life that take us out of ourselves. He calls this "self-less pleasure," as opposed to "self-based pleasure," which comes from a variety of pursuits of the flesh, such as sex, food, drink, and drugs. When our larger connection is with God, we trigger the biological mechanism for a joy that fulfills us. We experience "the something more" that is always left and longed for when we have our fill of self-based pleasure. We have not only joy but peace, and a sense of blessing.

Chapter Nine

BOUNCING BACK: AGAIN AND AGAIN

We have got to warm ourselves back to the certainty
that it is only when we lose the connection
between ourselves and other people
that we begin to freeze up in despair.

—MAY SARTON

R esilience is the ability to bounce back after suffering set-backs and losses, such as loss of physical health or free-dom from pain. We are more resilient if we are able to transform adversity into accomplishment, to use physical crisis as a challenge to grow emotionally and heal the nonphysical self—especially when curing the body is not possible.[1]

We have seen how the alchemy of metaphorically turning dross into gold is facilitated by our having gratitude, purpose, and faith, each of which enlarges and enriches our lives and lifts us beyond ourselves to something larger. The empirical and anecdotal evidence also clearly tells us that healthy bonding with others plays an essential role in whether we succeed in bouncing back after being laid low.

If we have a chronic, recurring disease or disability, rebounding isn't measured by our success in getting rid of the problem. If it's chronic or recurring, the condition is with us to stay, in either a latent or overt form. Depression is a recurring condition. So are cancer, heart disease, hypertension, stroke, and other leading causes of death and disability. Bouncing back for those of us who have one of these conditions is measured by the sense of being well inside ourselves—in other words, by the degree of inner health we hold onto or regain.

How successful we are at establishing and maintaining close, enduring relations with others, in good times and bad, is a major factor in both our resilience and our survival. A longitudinal study in Israel found that the effects of heart disease—such as hypertension and high cholesterol—could be "counteracted" if a husband felt he had his wife's love and support.[2] Recent longitutidinal studies involving thousands of people in 26 projects showed that "being married (or socially supported in other ways) was generally associated with survival" and recovery from serious illnesses, particularly coronary artery disease.[3]

FULFILLING THE NEED TO BOND

For where there is love of man, there is also love of the art. For some patients, though conscious that their condition is perilous, recover their health simply through their contentment with the goodness of their physician.

—HIPPOCRATES

The need to bond is so ingrained in the human psyche and soma that physicians who connect with patients are able to use it therapeutically.[4] As Suchman and Matthews (Chapter 3) suggested in describing the "connexional experience," these are doctors who recognize that "pain, loss of function, and other types of distress disrupt ordinary means of making contact, thus intensifying the isolation of everyday existence."[5]

Our resilience is enhanced by "a feeling of connectedness with the doctor, of being deeply heard and understood.... Wholly independent of whatever biotechnical treatment is offered, this deep, transpersonal connectedness between the patient and doctor...is comforting and therapeutic."[6] If we want to rebound as far as we can, physically and nonphysically, then we will select our doctor carefully. The connexional experience of physician and patient can be so strong that some seriously ill persons are known to "get well" for their doctor (see Dr. Carlos Peete, p. 170).[7]

EFFECTS OF GOOD TOUCHING

Touch me, touch the palm of your hand
to my body as I pass.
—WHITMAN

Physicians, nurses, and other health professionals also affect our physiological and psychological health by the positive touching they can provide our bodies. The evidence has been clear for some time that blood pressure decreases and heart rhythm stabilizes when sick people have their hands held or they are stroked in a caring way.[8] Dr. Tiffany Field, director of the Touch Research Institute at the University of Miami School of Medicine, and her colleagues have shown that premature infants gain weight faster when they are massaged regularly.[9]

When volunteer grandparents, many of whom had suffered losses of loved ones or had lost the social support that previously provided them with hugs and good touching, were trained to massage abused infants, both the young and old benefited.[10] The grandparents perked up psychologically from feeling needed and, because they were also given regular massages while volunteering, they enjoyed physical benefits as well.

LONGER AND BETTER LIFE

*Happy, thrice happy and more, are they whom
an unbroken bond unites and whose love shall know
no sundering quarrels so long as they shall live.*

—HORACE

The evidence is also clear that the more attached we are to others, the longer we will live. Whether we have heart disease or cancer, the two leading causes of death, our survival will be significantly increased if we have friends, good family relations, and a loving marriage.[11]

Ideally, our goal in being resilient is to live not only longer but better in the wake of withstanding a loss or setback—that is, to use the experience to enhance our quality of life even in the face of continued pain. When we suffer a recurrence, flareup, or bout of cancer, coronary artery disease, depression, or diabetes, we hope both to live through it and to retain a life worth living. The most resilient of the wounded but well deal with a relapse not only by using their pain or loss creatively to discover new ways to appreciate what's good in life, to enhance the purpose of their existence, and to strengthen their faith but also by knowing what not to do. They don't engage in self-pity, blame, cynicism, hostility, or envy. Refusing to engage in these behaviors not only allows for better bonding with others but for more freedom from the problems that make relationships conflictual and stressful.

In both young people and old, bonding is seen as the most highly valued activity or experience we can have. In a study of 108 college students and 109 persons 65 years or older, researchers at Kent State University recently found that "interacting with friends and family" was rated as "the most valued life activity."[12] Any condition that makes bonding virtually impossible—such as inability to reason, remember, communicate—was considered by both groups as "fates worse than death."

The quality of our life is largely shaped not by physical health but by the "web of relationships with self and others."[13] Lasting, intimate bonding with at least one other person in our life plus committed connections with groups gives us strength to persevere.[14]

Lasting survival of institutions, as well as people, depends on bonding. The noted Harvard sociologist Pitirim Sorokin made a study of standing institutions across millennia and found that religions based on love, altruism, and bonding have survived longer than all others.[15] The fact that love heals, if not cures, has been well-established.[16] Bonding and love are such healers because they enlarge us and take us beyond ego and the physical self. They "increase" the nonphysical self, as we suggested in Chapter 2.

TWO SIDES OF LOVE

Love is most nearly itself when
here and now cease to matter.

—T. S. ELIOT

What has been less recognized are the two sides of love, one having to do with giving and the other with receiving. Love is often talked about as something to give, with little said of the grace to receive. "The experience of love is not unilateral. To experience the fullness of love," we must know how to accept as well as give.[17]

I have known people who struggled mightily with illness, particularly recurring illness, largely because they have such trouble receiving love and help from others. They are good at only one-way love, which allows them to do all the giving (see Lawlis in Chapter 3). Resilience requires two-way love, which means that we recognize the need of another person to give love to us. The ability to accept it comfortably may have to be developed. In Fryback's study of health in people with terminal diseases (see Chapter 1), those interviewed agreed that the ability both to give and to receive love was necessary for a sense of health. Families often need and want to take care of a dying parent or loved one at home.

Eileen Reed, a breast cancer survivor whom we will meet again later in this chapter, said: "The hardest part of the last year was being dependent, having to ask for help or graciously know how to accept it. I have reassessed my life and how to accept love and help from others."[18]

ATTACHMENTS TO PETS AND PLANTS

Who loves me will love my dog also.

—ST. BERNARD OF CLAIRVAUX

We bond not only with other humans but with fauna and flora. A number of years ago, when I first wrote on this subject, the evidence was just emerging on the healing effects of having pets and plants. Because pets can provide a source of support, love, or companionship, research has shown that when people are hospitalized with heart attacks, their survival rates increase if they have an animal waiting for them at home.[19]

Katie (Chapter 3), who went through the crisis of being diagnosed with breast cancer and undergoing surgery and chemotherapy while pregnant, has houseplants and a whole pack of pets to encourage her resilience. They help her feel needed. In addition to her little girl and husband, she has eight cats, a rabbit, a bird, a dog, and fish. "They are a calming influence," Katie said. When she is upset or angry, she finds herself petting the cats and forgets why she was mad. When she feels lonely, she talks to her animals, particularly to the Siamese cat, which talks back, she reports. Katie grew up on a farm and has bonded with animals since she was a child. She and her family still live in the country.

Katie has benefited not only from the support her animals offer but also from the sense of responsibility she has toward them. "I've always liked having responsibility," she said. She has long taken care of sick animals she finds. Research has shown that when residents in nursing homes are given potted plants and are asked to take care of them, these people have less illness and live longer.[20] When we feel we are needed, then, we are more likely to be resilient.

My bonding with animals goes back to early childhood, when my parents brought a dog named "Rags" home and later agreed that my brother and I could add a second canine we named "Sport." I played with these dogs in the backyard in all kinds of weather and in all kinds of ways, including, when I was just a toddler, sitting in the big Number 2 washtub with Rags while he got his bath. Both these dogs lived long past their life expectancy. Rita and I had the same experience with Snoopy, part dachshund, part terrier, who lived for 19 years. His fearlessness and tenacity saw him through long runs and mountain hikes, where his low center of gravity was a great benefit and his legs were just long enough to give him strength and speed. When Snoopy got stem cell cancer, I thought he was gone. But radiation therapy kept him on his feet until finally he was hit by a car. He was so loved and known by neighbors that 35 people attended a memorial service in our back-yard, where we buried part of his ashes. The remaining ashes we scattered among big boulders he had climbed in the Rockies.

Today we have Tashi, who is Tibetan—at least genetically he is. We tested the authenticity of his Himalayan Mountain genes when he was 4 months old by taking him on a climb in the mountains and snow. He took to both as though he was home, which he was, in a sense. We like to think that Tashi (whose name in Tibetan means "auspicious" or "audacious," depending on the translation) also has genes for mindfulness, which his ancestors had to demonstrate in order to be the watchdogs and pets of the Tibetan monks high in the Himalayas. As if from some ancient wisdom, he knows when to lie down and be quiet during meditation time, which enhances our bonding. I agree with Audrey Ronning Topping, who wrote of her family's 30 years with a remarkable cockatoo named Charlie, that "we are all one with nature and all God's creatures. We are all in this great adventure together."[21]

OUTLOOK COUNTS MORE THAN GENES

As you grow older, you evolve from body to mind to spirit, and as you let go of once supreme pleasures, you discover even finer new pleasures.

—GEORGE SHEEHAN

Love and bonding are ingredients in successful aging, which chronic disease or disability often challenges. Both depend on staying involved with others, identifying new goals to meet and projects to complete, having a feeling of being needed and a sense of being effective, and remaining active physically as much as the body permits.

Helen Page is as an example.[22] At 83, she "has never let anything get her down for long." At one time or another she has had a broken neck from an automobile accident, breast cancer, and two heart attacks. The former schoolteacher is a near vegetarian who drinks a glass of wine before dinner and walks two miles before breakfast. A model of bonding behavior, Ms. Page has "astronomical" phone bills "from the calls I make trying to encourage friends to keep going when things are bad."[23] She believes she should do something good for someone else each day.

Because research findings now suggest that "people are largely responsible for their own old age"—meaning that good health habits and an optimistic outlook on life count more than the influence of genes—we can realistically retain a degree of control over our lives as we get older. Contrary to earlier impressions, PET scans and magnetic resonance imaging studies show that the brain does not shrink with age as much as had been thought.[24] The shrinkage that does occur fails to result in any significant loss in cognitive abilities. The National Long Term Care Survey, which tracks the health of almost 20,000 persons 65 and older, revealed that "every year there is a smaller and smaller percentage of old people who are unable to take care of themselves, unable to comb their hair, feed themselves, or take a walk."[25] There were 121,000 fewer disabled persons in 1995 than in 1992 among those from 65 to 74 years old. As people assume more responsibility for their health and place less emphasis on the role of genes, they lower the risk of disability from disease.

Studies begun in 1985 funded by the MacArthur Foundation on successful aging have found that genes count most early in life in affecting our health characteristics. By age 80, "for many of the characteristics there is hardly any genetic influence left," according to a member of the research team, Dr. Gerald E. McClearn, a gerontological geneticist at Pennsylvania State University.[26] It is true that aches and pains are more frequent as we age and the risk of chronic disease increases, but when sickness occurs for those who have kept physically, socially, and mentally active, rebounding comes easier.

RESILIENCE IN LATER LIFE

If wrinkles must be written upon our brows,
let them not be written upon the heart.
The spirit should not grow old.

—JAMES A. GARFIELD

Old age challenges not only our resilience but our mental acumen. Although brain shrinkage is not significant in the elderly, decline in episodic memory—memory for where we had lunch last week or what we read two nights ago—will occur if we don't keep novelty, new experiences, and other forms of stimulation in our lives.[27] Some sense of control and a feeling of being needed also are important.

The most resilient older person I know is a lifelong family friend, Violet Gilbert, 99, of Dallas, who still reads voluminously, is full of questions about events, from local to international, does daily exercises, and assists her daughter, Gloria, who was stricken years ago by polio. Her exercises consist of sit ups, leg lifts, forward bends, and shoulder rotations. Violet was my mother's best friend until my mother died at age 92. She and Violet had known each other since both my parents met at the home of Violet's family in East Dallas shortly after World War I.

Violet was more than 85 when she shuttered her own house, where she had lived 60 years or so, and moved in with her daughter, Gloria, to assume caretaking duties. Gloria, whose husband had suffered a fatal heart attack, needed help because she was struck down by polio more than 40 years ago when she was a vivacious, young woman who loved to jitterbug. Now she was confined to a wheelchair and had suffered broken bones from falls. Violet has had years of experience in the caretaking role. Her own husband had died after a lingering illness, and one by one she ministered to a number of her brothers and sisters as they got older, became sick, and died. Violet has continued to drive her own car, recover quickly from her own illnesses, do all she could to relieve pain from hammertoes and swollen feet, maintain a network of friends through church and community activities, and acquire great-grandchildren and great-great grandchildren. In March 1996 she became seriously dehydrated, was admitted to intensive care in a hospital, finally diagnosed with acute myelomonocytic leukemia, and nearly died.

During the time she was critically ill, I talked with her one day by phone. With labored breath, she told me, "This comes to everyone. I'll be 98 in a few months if I live. If I don't, that's okay, I'm ready to go. I've helped others all my life. There are still ones who need me, but if it's time for me to go, that's okay." She thanked me and Rita for keeping up with her and spending time with her each time we went to Dallas. "I love you for all you have done for me. Now I must say good-bye." She hung up, and I thought that would be the last time I would talk with her. I was wrong. She not only recovered and regained most of her stamina but within a few months was also dancing the Marcarena at a wedding reception her great-niece took her to.

Violet continues to have sharp long-term and short-term memory, extraordinary eyesight, and hearing for her age, and an enthusiasm for life based on delight in the ordinary, curiosity, and a desire to learn and be of help to others. She credits her vitality to enjoyment of people, good food and music, the beauty of nature, and the value of prayer, which she used repeatedly when there were doubts she would recover. Her goal is to start driving again, so she will have a way to go to church, and to live to at least 100.

When we visited her a few months after she got out of the hospital at Gloria's home, where she has resumed her caretaking role, she proudly showed us a new T-shirt she had been given, which had emblazoned on the front: "Genuine All-American Antique Person—Been There, Done That. I'm History." She is a living history of perseverance.

Violet again demonstrated her resilience nine months later when she broke her right hip. At 1:30 AM she was feeding her usual inquisitiveness by reading every line in the newspaper when she nodded off and fell from her chair at the kitchen table to the floor. The doctor who did her surgery said she was the oldest person he had ever operated on. It went well, and within two days Violet was saying she was ready to "get on with going on." At her bedside when we visited her was a vase of lavender irises from her son, who grew them from a root stock of irises in Violet's own yard. If life is like a plant that lives on its rhizome, as Jung believed (see Chapter 7), then Violet has a lot of life left in her.[28]

<hr>

STORIES THAT GIVE US REASONS TO BOUNCE BACK

Setting goals and having positive expectations about reaching them significantly influence our capacity to retain a sense of well-being during a severe illness or a long-term course of medical treatment requiring powerful drugs. Violet has little doubt she will be walking when she is 100. Studies show that patients in pain who strongly expect their future health to be better rate their present health positively, regardless of their medical status.[29] People's "expectancies for the future," researchers found, have to be understood to account for the ratings they give their own health.[30] Positive expectations, in turn, are related to establishing goals that keep us committed. Goals often grow out of the stories we tell ourselves about our lives that give meaning to them.

Jeff Getty, an AIDS patient and activist in California, made medical history when he received, at age 38, an infusion of bone marrow cells from a baboon. Taking such a risk was consistent with his story. He saw himself as "a soldier in the front lines of AIDS, someone willing to die for the cause if necessary, someone willing to take chances."[31] A year after the first simian-to-human bone marrow transplant ever, Getty was not only alive but had gained 20 pounds and was feeling better than he had in five years.

Robert Massie's story is different. He has attracted medical and media attention by his resistance to AIDS for 20 years without any drug therapy. A hemophiliac, Massie, 41, was infected with what became known as the human immunodeficiency virus—apparently through a tainted blood transfusion—even before AIDS was recognized as a disease and HIV identified as the agent. "I have a tremendous sense of gratitude," he said.[32] Acutely conscious of time being given back to him after he feared it had been taken away, he is committed to "using my time wisely." Massie, an Episcopal priest, now directs a national environmental group.

Countless other AIDS resisters and survivors have shown a quieter power of positive expectations in contradicting the early, widespread belief that AIDS is invariably fatal and HIV infection means full-blown symptoms will occur in time. Many of those with AIDS and positive HIV tests have now gone for years without such outcomes. Strong social support, exercise, meditation, imagery, and avoidance of street drugs have been credited with maintaining immune competence.[33]

ADVENTURES TO ENLIVEN US

Chasing yesterday is a bad show.
You don't want to live backwards.

—HEMINGWAY

In recurrent disease, where remission comes and goes, those who hold on to their inner health find new adventures and challenges to enliven and energize them. At 77, after undergoing not only chemotherapy and hormonal therapy for metastatic prostate cancer but also later suffering a heart attack, Max Lerner (Chapter 3) was offered a university professorship by Notre Dame. He loved to teach but he had to be physically able to go to Notre Dame. Lerner not only became well enough to accept the Notre Dame offer but, until he was 89, when he died, he continued to write a newspaper column on world events twice a week. Up to two years before then, his son Michael notes, "he flew regularly from New York to California to teach a course at one of the few universities that does not discriminate against vibrantly alive 87-year-old men."[34] In 1990, Max Lerner's acclaimed book *Wrestling with the Angel,* on his experience with cancer and heart disease, was published, another testimony to his resilience.

Resilience often depends on our having an enthusiasm—literally, a god within—for life, which in turn depends on our seeing life as an adventure. Max Lerner had such enthusiasm. In working with cancer patients, psychologist Lawrence LeShan asks them: "What kind of life would make you glad to get up in the morning and go to bed at night 'good tired?' What would give you the maximum zest and enthusiasm in life?"[35] Whatever brings color and feeling into our life not only quickens the spirit but enhances immune function.[36]

TAKING DELIGHT IN THE ORDINARY

If we had a keen vision of all that is ordinary in human life, it would be like hearing the grass grow or the squirrel's heart beat. . . .

—GEORGE ELIOT

Adventures and challenges come in smaller sizes as well as larger ones. After Mrs. A, a 51-year-old editor at a New York fashion magazine, was diagnosed with metastatic breast cancer, she bought an apple orchard in the country and set out to build a house there as a place to spend long weekends.[37] The project became an adventure for her, and following one particular weekend, she came in to the office of her psychotherapist "buoyant." Mrs. A had "found a spot in the orchard where she could see the entire vista of her property, and, seated there because she could hardly stand, she noticed the arrival of a flock of bluebirds."[38] For hours she watched the birds build their nests, which gave her such joy she told her therapist, "I had the greatest weekend!"

Taking delight in the ordinary adds small drama to our lives when we are limited physically but not spiritually or emotionally. "The minutiae of my life have had to assume dramatic proportions," observed author Nancy Mairs in her struggles with multiple sclerosis and depression.[39] "If I could not . . . delight in them, they would likely throw me into rage and self-pity."

Mairs discovered she could turn "minutiae" into adventure: ". . . whether I am feeding fish flakes to my bettas . . . lying wide-eyed in the dark battling yet another bout of depression, cooking a chicken. . . . I am always having the adventures that are mine to have."[40]

Both Mrs. A with her orchard and bluebirds and Nancy Mairs with her small delights added excitement to daily existence with their ventures of the spirit and imagination. They also made a challenge out of their adversity. Mrs. A took on building a house in the country. Mairs learned to look upon just buttoning her shirt, changing a light bulb, and walking down stairs as challenges, which result in "a lift of the spirit" when accomplished.

When Katie (Chapter 3) was faced with being told by oncologists that she was only the thirteenth patient they knew of who was being treated for breast cancer while pregnant, she was also informed that the surgery she needed might cause a spontaneous abortion. She had already made the decision not to have an abortion despite her cancer diagnosis and treatment. Katie took all this on as a challenge. "When people tell me I can't do something, then I do it." What she did in this case was both to undergo the surgery successfully and give birth to a healthy baby girl.

In a study in Milan, Italy, of 25 persons who had become blind as adults and 20 persons who had become paraplegic, the most resilient were those who accepted everything as a new how-to challenge: how to get around a room, how to dress, how to eat.[41] Instead of taking life for granted, as they had before their misfortune, "now every little thing they accomplished made them feel good. They had to plan. They had to develop a skill to do things."[42] Instead of seeing this as a burden, "They seemed to feel that if they worked hard they could always improve. Somehow that effort and success boosted their self-confidence tremendously."[43]

"A Proud and Joyous Moment"

What is harder than rock, or softer than water?
Yet soft water hollows out hard rock. Persevere.

—OVID

Eileen Reed, 66, who learned about accepting love, had to have challenge thrust upon her to awaken her latent resilience. After a mastectomy and a round of chemotherapy ending in December 1995, she set out to regain the strength she had as a runner and skier. But plastic surgery and a hernia operation eliminated skiing for the season and she didn't have the stamina to resume running. She tried some hiking in Scotland, but, without energy, she gave it up despite a yearning to feel well again and participate in sports.

A few weeks later, her support group volunteered her in her absence to join three others in the group to enter a triathlon sponsored by an aerobic clothing manufacturer. With only two months before the triathlon, it acted "like a kick in the butt" to Eileen.[44] "I had to show those young 'uns that we can still do it," she said. The triathlon involved a half-mile swim in a lake, a 12-mile bike ride and a 3.1 mile walk or run. She resumed her running and bike riding and enlisted the support of a woman who taught her how to swim in six weeks.'

"It was a proud and joyous moment" when she and her two team members, also cancer survivors, "marched arm in arm across the finish line" at the triathlon. Eileen finished first in her age group. She said: "I am not the same person I was a year and a half ago. I have a new self-image that is different. I am stronger because I have been through the fire."[45]

KEEPING ON KEEPING ON

Over the last 10 years, Wilfred Tapper, now 80, has had—in chronological order—four surgeries for Graves' Disease, five weeks of radiation for prostate cancer, an emergency abdominal operation for a perforated ulcer, and physical therapy for muscular dystrophy, which was diagnosed in 1993. He has never asked "Why me?" questions or whether life is worthwhile when one is besieged by serious infirmities. He has a strong belief in the human capacity "to do what you have to do," which for him is to continue living so he can continue "accomplishing things."[46] Helping him do what he has to is Fannie Tapper, 70, his wife of 15 years, who has her own kind of resilience as one of the legion of spouses, mates, parents, and friends who "stand and wait" while the loved ones undergo painful procedures and treatment for life-threatening diseases. Instead of just waiting, she has done an outstanding serial photographic portrait of Wif and his long battle with diseases and disorders, which have yet failed to defeat him. "What you see over the span of time covered by the photos is a series of disasters," says Fannie Tapper.[47] "What I'm trying to show is how one person can go through all that and still come out with energy and optimism and willpower."

Each time before the orbital surgeries to save his vision, which was endangered by the Graves' Disease resulting from hyperthyroidism, Wif's doctors would test his heart and ask him: "How are you feeling?" He knew that they were asking him if he felt he could stand up to the surgery. "I can do it" was his response. Wif doesn't "keep on keeping on," as Fannie calls it, out of fear of dying but from the belief that he hasn't finished "accomplishing things." He has had a long career as an international consultant for major oil companies and other large corporations and still has plans to negotiate additional deals in the Middle East. "He believes he will be viable forever," Fannie says.

FOUR C'S OF RESILIENCE

You can hold yourself back from suffering . . .
but perhaps precisely this holding back is the only
suffering you might be able to avoid.

—KAFKA

When we come out of adversity with greater inner strength we add to our semblance of control in life. We have the feeling, as many in our cancer study reported, that if we can handle what once seemed too much for us, then we can deal with most anything. Challenge and control, combined with commitment to pursuits larger than the self, constitute three C's that make for hardiness, a well-researched attribute that enhances not only health but resilience.[48]

A fourth C that contributes to our durability is courage (see Chapters 3 and 6), both the courage to dare and the courage to endure, to take risks and to show fortitude. What we often associate courage with in illness is withstanding pain or undergoing aggressive surgical and medical treatment that produces powerful side-effects. Patients often feel or are told they are in a fierce battle and they must fight back like a warrior. I agree there are circumstances requiring such an active stance, but no less heroic is the courage to resist trying so hard that we break the connection with the sources of our core health. When we try to grasp a beautiful butterfly resting in the palm of our hand, we crush it. "To entice it to remain there, you must make the nectar of your life so sweet that the butterfly. . . is irresistibly drawn to stay."[49]

There is yet another kind of courage that resilience requires. This is the courage to confront ourselves on what we find too painful or shameful to acknowledge in ourselves or what we don't want others to know about us. Whatever our dark side is, it takes courage to deal with it, and we can't overcome loss and failures with resilience until we do.

The research of Dr. James Pennebaker, longtime professor of psychology at Southern Methodist University now at the University of Texas in Austin, has shown the benefits of self-confrontation and disclosure in both sickness and health.[50] He and other researchers have found that talking or writing about traumatic experiences, including shameful ones, improves immune function, reduces visits to physicians for illness, and brings better performance at work or school.[51] Pennebaker himself discovered how his own unacknowledged feelings were an underlying cause of his asthma attacks. He would have bouts of wheezing when he went home to West Texas to visit his parents for the Christmas holidays but attributed the problem to the pollen and dust blown in from New Mexico and Nevada. He was forced to look deeper when one November his parents came to visit him in Florida, a region clearly free of blowing dust and West Texas pollen. "The day they arrived I developed asthma. All of a sudden, the profound realization hit me that there was more to asthma than pollen. Conflicts with my parents were undoubtedly linked to my upper respiratory system."[52] After Pennebaker confronted his submerged feelings and "saw the parent-asthma connection, I never again wheezed."

ESCAPING INSTEAD OF FACING

The past is not a package one can lay away.
—EMILY DICKINSON

Confronting personal issues related to self also may require facing up to whether we are using religion or spirituality to avoid self-examination of our deep psychological issues. Feeling connected to God and transcending the self will not automatically free us from emotional baggage we prefer not to face. In fact, as Dr. Frances Vaughan has observed, spirituality and religion can be used as an escape from dealing with repressed feelings and psychic pain.[53] If we don't deal with them, we will have only limited success at recovery and very little resilience. We may rebound once or twice but not repeatedly. Eventually, the baggage becomes too heavy for us to carry any longer.

The women I mentioned earlier who finally faced up to the sexual abuse they suffered as children at the hands of their fathers remarkably diminished their pain as cancer patients and lightened their lives (see Dorothy in Chapter 4 and 6 and Ellen in Chapter 6). Gay Robertson (also Chapter 6) started working on unloading her psychic pain from abuse even before she suffered serious heart problems. Several women in our cancer study had to own up to bad marriages and leave corrosive relationships as part of their recovery. Deanna (Chapter 7) was confronted with being abandoned by her husband when she was diagnosed with cancer. He barely got to the hospital once to see her during the two weeks she was there the first time. He was long gone by the time of her metastases. Lilly had to face up to her husband's and best friend's infidelity (Chapter 2). Sandy (Chapter 6) found out after she was diagnosed with cancer that her husband was seeing another woman and wanted a divorce. She had to confront her own depression and fantasy that he would change his mind. Dana (Chapter 2) tried marriage early, but when it failed she decided to build her close relations around friends, pets, and flowers.

Until we dump the baggage of suppressed secrets, shame, and failures, it will drag us down with hidden fear, anxiety, and anger. For many years I could not openly admit that I had a schizophrenic son who was locked up in the maximum security unit of a state hospital. I compensated by focusing on the accomplishments of our daughter Cindy, who overcame her own stressful childhood to graduate from medical school and become a board-certified internist. I also used to talk readily of Liz's days at boarding school, her study of art in France and Spain, her graduation in long white dress, broadbrim straw hat, and elbow length gloves, while the sounds of Pachelbel's Canon in D played in the background. But all that changed.

After her—and my—house of cards crumbled, I went underground with the pain of her ensuing years as a drug addict on the streets of Manhattan and the repeated failures of drug treatment programs she entered. My "coming out" occurred only when I came face to face with the fact that my own deepening depression would not ease until, as I said earlier, I acknowledged her impending death as well as my own mortality and start doing something to prepare for both (see Chapters 2, 4, and 5).

It is action, beyond meditation, prayer, and belief in a larger life, that repeated resilience also requires. Freud as well as Marx insisted that religion is an opiate people use to relieve pain they refuse to acknowledge or act upon. Religion does give comfort and offer a refuge from pain, but it should facilitate, not preclude, taking concrete steps in the very real, everyday world to cope with fears and failures and to let go of shame.

CONFRONTING THE DARKEST SIDE

Two Episcopal preachers have impressed me with their self-confrontation and ability to rebound from loss and failure. Both had to face their own kind of grandiosity. In a story that made headlines in the newspapers of New Orleans, Rev. John Jenkins, the popular rector of a well-established Garden District Anglican church, was "scandalized" by the death of his alcoholic wife, killed at home in a struggle with their grown son.[54]

Filled with pain and shame Jenkins sat in the back pew on the first Sunday he returned to the church after the terrible event. A man who took great pride in his self-sufficiency, Jenkins now needed acceptance and support more than he had ever acknowledged needing either before. His congregation rallied behind him, and those at the Sunday service insisted he come up front and assume his usual position behind the altar rail. He confessed he had not been a good husband and asked forgiveness.

Jenkins later got a second chance at marriage—"a gift from God"—and set out to be an attentive, loving husband to his new wife. After leaving New Orleans, he found himself in demand on the workshop circuit giving talks and sermons at churches on coping with acute psychological pain and dealing with unexpected loss and shame. He retained, even strengthened his faith in Jesus Christ, but never hesitated to say that religion is not meant to suppress strong human emotion, even rage, when one spouse betrays another, when an innocent child suffers a painful death, when a good person is dealt only bad hands.

Confronting our deepest and most unacknowledged feelings and the darkest side of our souls is the starting point if recovery is to lead to resilience. When religion becomes a refuge from confrontation with ourselves, undealt-with psychological issues will eventually cripple us not only emotionally but spiritually. Reverend John Claypool found that when bad things happen to good people we often need to be confronted with the reality that all of us, good, bad, and indifferent, get rained on sooner or later, and even the best may find themselves mired in mud.[55] Despite the best of medical science and the most fervent of prayers, Claypool and his wife lost their 8½-year-old daughter to acute lymphatic leukemia.

Some time later, a rabbi friend stopped Claypool in the lobby of the hospital where his little girl had died and asked him: "Did God do anything for any of you through all of this?" Claypool took a long time to answer, since their pleas for a miracle and for a medical solution had gone unanswered and he had asked himself the same question. Then it became clear to him what God had done. "He gave me the ability to endure," he answered his friend.

Later Claypool's marriage failed. His wife told him she no longer wanted to continue their relationship of more than 20 years. Stunned by all that had happened Claypool moved away, full of replays of the past and "if only" ruminations. He had witnessed many painful events happening to others, and was always there to help, but out of his own grandiosity, he never thought such failure and loss could occur in his own life. He entered psychotherapy and in the course of it was in effect asked, "What makes you so special to believe that you should be exempt from such pain or be so gifted as to avoid it?" The second question was, "When are you going to join the human race?" The confrontation produced an awakening, which led to Claypool's "joining the human race," and recovery began.

An often quoted passage from *Isaiah*[56]—a favorite of marathon runners hitting the proverbial wall—promises that God will give the faithful the strength to mount up as if on wings of eagles, to run and not be weary. The last part of the passage is the verse Claypool, and many of us, can best identify with and appreciate most: God also gives us the strength, if we have faith, just to walk without fainting. Sometimes that is all it takes to be resilient.

In the next and final chapter, we will see how even the time of our dying presents us with the opportunity to repair ourselves, to claim our health, and to quicken the spirit.

Chapter Ten

DYING

WELL

Write the wrongs that are done to you on sand, but write the good things that happen to you on a piece of marble. Let go of all emotions such as resentment and retaliation, which diminish you, and hold onto the emotions, such as gratitude and joy, which increase you.

—ARAB PROVERB

I f sick persons can have a different kind of health, they also can die well. Dying well means we die healed—healed in two senses: (1) that we have made peace with ourselves, our God, and others; (2) that we have experienced losing the self in something larger and have gained spirit.

Inner peace is such a built-in, "hard-wired" need that it must have something to do with defining who we are and what it means to be a human being. We want peace not only at death but in life. When we have peace, we experience it at our core level, in our spirit. It defines our human essence. Dom Laurence Freeman, who teaches groups around the world the ways of living and dying better, sees peace in terms of what it is and isn't.

> Peace is not just peace of mind. It is not just control of pain. Peace is a reality of the whole person and therefore a spiritual reality. It is an energy. It isn't just being calm. It isn't just being protected from worry or anxiety. . . . This energy is . . . something that arises from the center of the human person. . . . We can be in the long-desired situation, the long-awaited environment and still lack peace. We have to be at peace with our selves if we are to be peaceful.[1]

If the peace we need is from repairing relationships with other people, we can do that ahead of dying or, given enough time, even in the process of dying. Whereas curing is bestowed on us from the outside and is not always possible, healing comes from inside and is almost always available. What we can heal are resentments, disappointments, anger, bitterness, memories, and anything else that goes into broken relationships that need repair.[2] What it takes—especially in healing our relationships with others—is swallowing our pride, giving up our demands that life treat us fairly, admitting we were hurt by someone, acknowledging that we are more sensitive to criticism, thoughtlessness, and ingratitude than we like to believe we are.[3] In short, it requires letting go of our ego, which is constantly on alert to defend our self-importance and entrenched positions, if not our perceived infallibility.

WHY MAKE PEACE?

If we do not have peace within

ourselves, it is in vain to seek

it from outward sources.

—LA ROCHEFOUCAULD

It isn't easy letting our defenses down and forgiving the past. This is true because the persons who—in fact or fantasy—did us wrong and treated us badly are often our parents, siblings, friends, spouse, or children.[4] Why do it, then, if we are going to die anyway? Three reasons: (1) peace with self is impossible without peace with others; (2) peace makes dying easier and less painful; (3) peace is not only for us but for those we love who survive us.

The first step toward peace-making often comes with being more open with positive feelings, because the peace we usually need to make is with people close to us that we care about but who hurt us. It may involve breaking a longstanding habit of never saying "I love you" for fear of making ourselves vulnerable to even more hurt. Psychologist Lawrence LeShan (Chapter 9) tells of a man who came in for consultation when his mother was dying of cancer in a hospital. Son and mother had never been able to talk about feelings, good or bad, with one another. Now the son wanted to "relate to her more and somehow help her more at this parting time, but he had no idea as to how to go about this. The daily visits were becoming more and more dreary and depressing times in which they sat and looked at one another, held hands with nothing to say, and felt increasingly frustrated."[5]

Since the man knew very little about his mother's childhood, LeShan suggested he ask what her early years had been like, what the most exciting period of her whole life was, what was the best major decision she had made, as well as the worst. "In short, who was she and what life had she led?"

The man went back to his mother and said, "Because I love you and there is so much I don't know about you, I want to know about your life. . . ."[6] With the son's disclosure, the mother opened up, and the visits took on a warmth and depth new to both of them. "As they exchanged ideas and memories, both felt richer," LeShan said. "She became more and more interested, not only in telling him about her life but in exploring it for herself. Frequently she would say things about her own life such as 'I never thought of it in that way before' or 'So that was what that was all about.'" The mother's depressed, dispirited demeanor lightened. She had fewer complaints about the food, the doctors, the nurses. "Rather she had an active and excited sense of exploration."

One day the mother asked her son to leave a tape recorder with her overnight. She taped a message to him that she wanted him to play after her death. Five hours before she died, the woman changed even more. "She seemed to light up from within," the son said. "She became very calm and serene. Yes, that's the word, serene." She told her nurse she didn't need her usual pain medication. "She was calm, relaxed, and seemed somehow happier than I have ever seen her," her son reported.

The mother said good-bye, gave him a few messages to relay of forgiveness, peace, and good wishes for relatives and friends, then closed her eyes and died. The night before her funeral, the son played the message she had recorded for him. In it, she gave him thanks and gratitude for changing her "whole dying experience."[7] LeShan said "she died a transcendent death. The family was left with as little emotional scarring as possible."[8]

Dying a "transcendent death" means we get beyond the ego so we can forgive, make peace, and see our life from a larger perspective, which brings a sense of meaning. "We cannot really say good-bye to something without knowing what it was," LeShan observes. "Trying to give up, say farewell to, renounce our lives before fully accepting them, tends to lead to a death that is bitter and sad."[9]

WHY STORIES HEAL

No story is the same to us after the lapse of time . . . we . . . are no longer the same interpreters.

—GEORGE ELIOT

When we see that there is a pattern and meaning in the life we have lived, it is an exciting discovery that quickens the spirit and makes the time of dying a great, last adventure, a time of growth and healing. Dr. Ira Byock, president of the American Academy of Hospice and Palliative Medicine, makes this point about the power of stories:

Stories are the only satisfying way I know of exploring the paradox that people can become stronger and more whole as physical weakness becomes overwhelming and life itself wanes. The stories of patients and their families... show us how we can grow stronger within ourselves and closer to those we love as we confront the challenges of dying with honesty, caring and commitment.[10]

Stories are healing because they often reveal a core meaning to our lives, an essential truth about us, and meaning gives us strength. If our stories are listened to by others, it means we matter, and when we feel we matter and are listened to, we are not lonely and suffer less.[11] In escaping loneliness, we overcome one of the most common barriers to dying well.

When resentments and past wrongs are redressed, forgiveness exchanged, and relationships repaired, we die strong in the belief that we are truly members of one another, as the disciple Paul put it.[12] When we reconnect with others by telling our stories and opening our hearts, we are brought closer together and experience not only peace but joy.[13]

TWO FOREMOST FEARS

For it is better to die of hunger,
so that you be free from pain and fear,
than to live in plenty and be troubled in mind.
—EPICTETUS

Dying alone and dying painfully are two foremost fears that many people have about death, and they clearly preclude dying well. As a young medical student, Frances Sharkey had had no experience with death until she was assigned her first patient at a large city hospital.[14] Her patient turned out to be a 92-year-old woman dying of heart failure who had once been an artist's model so celebrated that her portrait still hung at the Metropolitan Museum of Art. "I studied her face, looking for traces of the beauty that had once been there," Sharkey said.[15] "I longed to ask her about her life," about what it was like to be beautiful and sought after when young, to work with great artists, and now to be alone and dying. But the story was too long and the patient too weak. She also was afraid. She could only gasp: "Don't leave me." So Sharkey sat holding the woman's hand long hours after her fellow medical students had left the hospital.

The woman would occasionally open her eyes and look at Sharkey as though wanting to talk. When the young student moved closer and looked at her face, the woman managed a faint smile. "What could she be thinking?" Sharkey wondered... "What did death feel like as it approached? Could she possibly tell me?" Sharkey removed the woman's oxygen mask and bent close to her, asking, "What is it like?" There was a long pause as though the patient hadn't heard the question. But finally, the old woman answered in a weak voice, "It's hard. Very hard."

To die well is not always possible, but enough is known now about what makes for a "good death" to emphasize that it is important to use the process of dying to resolve and complete relationships.[16] In Dr. Byock's experience, "Patients who died most peacefully and families who felt enriched by the passing of a loved one tended to be particularly active in terms of their relationships and discussions of personal and spiritual matters."[17] Physical pain, hospice physicians insist, can be controlled, but relief of emotional suffering depends on a good relationship with loved ones and God.

THE WAY WE DIE

As discussed in the chapter on faith, the evidence on prayer suggests that each of us can reach beyond the body, that who we are is something more than matter, and that although the body dies, our essence, our spirit does not. When we understand this, we die in "perfect health."[18] Charles Meyer, who has been at the bedside of many dying patients as a hospital and hospice chaplain, sees the form that final healing often takes is death itself. "Death . . . is part of that ongoing process of healing, which ultimately results in being in 'God's nearer presence,' where perfect wholeness has occurred."[19] A holy death has in it an experience of oneness with God.

Dr. Sherwin Nuland, the Yale surgeon who wrote *How We Die: Reflections on Life's Final Chapter,* holds that "the great majority of people do not leave life in a way they would choose."[20] For himself, he seeks to die with dignity, but "the conditions of my illness may not permit me to 'die well' or with any of the dignity we so optimistically seek."[21] He suggests that the way to die well is to live well, that "the dignity that we seek in dying must be found in the dignity with which we have lived our lives."[22]

Those who seek physician-assisted suicide often base their pursuit on the desire not only to die with dignity but to escape the state of helplessness and hopelessness they believe is the inevitable end. Ben Mattlin, a 33-year-old Harvard graduate who was born with a profound neuromuscular disability and is confined to a wheelchair, points out that "a state of helplessness and being terminally ill" are not the same thing. "I have lived my whole life in such a state, needing assistance for eating, bathing, using the toilet. The human thing to do is to help, not presume that my life isn't worth living."[23] In regard to the active assistance that Dr. Jack Kervorkian has given to dozens of suicides since 1990 Mattlin goes on to say:

> Kervorkian would argue that he is ending suffering for people with no options. Tell that to Stephen Hawking, the physicist who has advanced amyotrophic lateral sclerosis, writes best-selling books, travels around the world and divorced his wife to marry his nurse. To say someone has no options just because doctors are stumped is medical arrogance. Quality of life is determined by more than physical condition.[24]

DYING IS MORE THAN A MEDICAL EVENT

*Retire from the world
like a satisfied guest.*

—HORACE

I suggest that if we exercise the options of repairing what has been broken in our relationships with ourselves, God, and others, we will die healed even though the conditions of our illness bring indignity, pain, and suffering to the body. If we discover, through making peace and getting beyond the self, that in our deepest being, we have a health that is impervious to disease, then we will have joy, as well as peace, as we die healed.

The whole idea of dying healed or dying well "is foreign to many people, families, and patients as well as medical people," mostly because they have not considered that "dying can encompass more than solely physical pain and tragedy."[25] Perhaps most of all, dying encompasses our experience of the life we are giving up.

I want to say at the very end of my life, "I am satisfied." I have been able to say that at the end of other episodes and events—writing a book, finishing some research, running a marathon, completing a climb, teaching a course, performing a service, returning on vacation from seeing the ruins at Paestum, listening to the *Ave Verum,* lying down at night after a full day and reading *Job* and the poetry of Pablo Neruda.

When Rachel Naomi Remen got to the hospital just in time to see her mother, who was being taken upstairs for cardiac bypass surgery, the 84-year-old woman said: "Oh good! . . . You're here! There was something that I wanted to tell you. I wanted to be certain you knew that no matter what happens here, *I am satisfied* and I hope you will do whatever you can to be satisfied as well."[26] These were the last lucid words Remen heard from her mother, who had been a public health visiting nurse who sat around many kitchen tables telling healing stories.

Dying satisfied is one way of dying well.

"THE BEST YEAR"

"C. D." made the same discovery. At 30, C. D. had been a world-class athlete and member of the national Canadian ski team. He was successful in business and engaged to be married when he was diagnosed with a "widely disseminated germinal testicular tumor." Dr. Balfour Mount (Chapter 2) performed six hours of radical surgery on him, which produced a temporary remission. But within months C. D.'s disease progressed and he died slowly over the next year. Mount said: "He had always been a winner. Strong. Outgoing. Gracious. A champion from a family of competitive champions, he was now melting before the raging forces of the embryonal cell."[27]

A few days before he died, C. D. married his fiancée, Grace, and "said good-bye to those he loved."[28] He told each of them, "This last year has been the best year of my life." The best year? Mount was astounded. Watching his patient's striking physical deterioration and contrasting that with the young man's "repeated physical and intellectual triumphs" of the past, the doctor had trouble believing that his patient could say "this has been the best year of my life." How could this be? C. D.'s answer was that he had discovered a core spirit in himself and, according to Mount, had gained "a new awareness of the spiritual dimension of human existence. Physical agony had been transcended through a journey inward that came to be characterized by grace and a sense of growth that he had not known."[29]

However we make the journey inward to our center, by meditation, prayer, spiritual discovery, music, art, poetry, or nature, we lose the self and gain spirit. More specifically, the ego-self is what we lose. When I am caught up in Beethoven's Pastorale or Raphael's "School of Athens," I have no thoughts of self, time, or space. I experience being joined to something deep and universal, good and immutable. In winter, when Rita and I are doing a walking meditation on a snowy trek in the Rockies, I have my eyes and ears open, but the sights and profound silence of the mountains merge into my mantra and the repetitive sounds of our snowshoes sliding beneath our boots. Meditation takes us underneath the turbulent stream of perceptions, thoughts, feelings, fears, and fantasies of the mind to an experience of peace and equanimity, which is a source of strength in the workaday world.

PREPARING TO DIE WELL

Most of us have time to prepare for dying well. ". . .we can consciously work toward dying well the way pregnant mothers work toward birthing well."[30] Because we all are terminal from birth, we have ample opportunity to practice how we will meet the death of the physical self. We don't have to wait until our dying time. But most people do wait, even those of us with disease or disability that recurs and keeps pain a constant companion. For us, we have even more reason to think about our finitude and dying time. Our culture strongly resists the idea of death and treats it as a "highly toxic," almost taboo subject.[31] Death is treated as sign of "failure, either of the doctor or of the patient," an attitude "at odds with that of other cultures" and our own past. As Dr. Michael Lerner, founder and president of Commonweal, reminds us:

> In many cultures, dying is surrounded by rituals in which everyone participates. For many centuries in the West, this was also so. Death was often seen as the culmination of a life, and people gave great thought to how they might die well. It is possible in our culture to *detoxify death* by contemplating it, seeing what others have thought and said about it, and by giving ourselves time to be with it. In the face of sincere contemplation and prayer, the toxicity with which our culture has surrounded death often begins to dissolve.[32]

Physicians too were once concerned with *ars moriendi,* the art of dying "the best way possible, at peace with God."[33] Doctors used to be skilled in the art of medicine, which included making death "as tranquil as professional kindness could."[34] Now, as Nuland points out:

> Except in the too-few programs such as hospice, that part of the art is now mostly lost, replaced by the brilliance of rescue and,

unfortunately the all-too-common abandonment when rescue proves impossible."[35]

With a false faith and illusion that medical science and technology will soon be able to rescue us all, we have kept the subject of death from our children and our homes. Children grow into adults never having seen death or even attended a funeral. I saw dying in the home in which I grew up as a boy, as Nuland did in his family, but I didn't admit death to my consciousness until much later. My grandfather died in the living room, where my parents had moved in a hospital bed for him. He died holding a glass of milk my mother had given him. His mouth was cocked open and his head angled back on the pillow, with his eyes staring at the ceiling. I was later to see that death posture many times in hospice work. After I left home, my father died of a stroke on the back steps, and 20 years later my mother died of heart failure in the back bedroom in the arms of a loving black caregiver named Fairie.

Reminding ourselves of our own finitude helps us to "value time, relationships, and the potential in each moment"[36] throughout our life as well as encourages us to practice detaching from ego and attaching to something larger.

LETTING GO OF EGO

Many could forego heavy meals, a full wardrobe, a fine house; it is the ego that they cannot forego.

—GANDHI

Surrendering ego, John Main said, comes from practice in letting go—a form of nonphysical dying, which he called "our first death."[37] Letting go of our physical self is our "second death," which is made easier by practice in the first. Main, who joined the British Foreign Service after studying law at Trinity College in Dublin, became a Benedictine monk who "saw meditation as a way of self-knowledge and self-acceptance."[38] Knowledge and acceptance of the self consists of understanding that at the center of our being, our essence, is spirit, whose fruits are love, joy, and peace.[39]

For years Main taught meditation worldwide and used it in preparation for his own death in 1982. Meditation is one way we learn of the deep dimension to ourselves that transcends words, thoughts, and the investments of ego. Dom Laurence Freeman, who studied literature at Oxford, joined Main's Benedictine Community and has carried on the Christian tradition of meditation. He saw the value of the mantra for terminally ill persons by being with John Main at his death. Main's last major talk outside his monastery was on the dying of the ego in life as essential preparation for dying of the body at death.

> He was in pain as he spoke, and he was relieved after the talk when we drove back to the monastery to lay him down on his bed.... His dying was a wondrous manifestation of the spiritual dimension of humankind. It was as if he was being filled with life to a point the body could not contain it.... When you were with him during that process of his dying you felt you were in the realm of spirit. You experienced the peace of his total centredness, the peace that is an energy, not just rest. There was joy, too, in his presence.... There was also light, a spiritual light that gave an insight into reality deeper than words or thoughts.... You could see it as Father John became increasingly translucent.[40]

RADIANCE AT DEATH

Now more than ever seems it rich to die,

To cease upon the midnight with no pain.

—KEATS

I have been struck by a calmness and kind of radiance I have seen on the faces of some dying persons at hospice. It may come in the process of losing themselves in stories about their lives and in memories of what captivated them the most.

One 75-year-old woman, with metastasized breast cancer whose face had this calmness and glow, told me of all the traveling she had done since retiring from many years with the Internal Revenue Service. She relived her trips abroad with a quiet excitement, pausing only to take telephone calls from friends, some of whom had traveled with her. Life had become an adventure to her upon retirement. She never knew she was so full of curiosity about the world and had such appreciation for the natural beauty she had found in the Swiss and Italian Alps, the Mediterranean coast, and the fjords of Norway, which were her favorite place. She was dying with the great satisfaction of developing a part of her soul that had remained dormant for many working years.

After Swiss psychologist C. G. Jung (Chapter 7) had broken his foot and suffered a heart attack in 1944, he became critically ill. Near death, he experienced a stream of images he would never forget. Jung wrote that "it is impossible to convey the beauty and intensity of emotion during those visions. They were the most tremendous things I have ever experienced."[41] Jung recovered and retained those joyous inner images for 17 more years, returning actively to them in the weeks before he finally died in 1961. An editor friend visited him during his last days and went into his study.

There was Jung sitting completely within himself. You really felt that this man was in his inner world, completely contained in his inner images; but then he realized that I was there. He turned round to me and his expression had changed. There was a man suddenly, utterly related to me. These two things, the immense concentration on his inner world and the immediate response to the other person, were to me the synthesis of the whole man.[42]

Jung, almost 86 years old, died "in great peace after a short illness at his house in Kusnacht.[43] The Latin inscription on his tombstone in the local cemetery reads:

VOCATUS ATQUE NON VOCATUS DEUS ADERIT
PRIMUS HOMO DE TERRA TERRENUS
SECUNDUS HOMO DE CAELO CAELESTIS.

It is from *I Corinthians,* Chapter 15, verse 47, which says: "The first man was of the dust of the earth, the second man from heaven." The two verses that follow tell us that "As was the earthly man, so are those who are of the earth; and as is the man from heaven, so also are those who are of heaven. And just as we have borne the likeness of the earthly man, so shall we bear the likeness of the man from heaven."[44]

Just as Jung lost himself in images of a deeper reality, many of which represented the universal archetypes and symbols he had studied for years, we have seen that others such as Madame Boulanger (Chapter 7) die with music in their heads and hearts. I would like to have for my dying time images of mountaintops, music of the masters, and the voices of those I love. If our Tibetan dog, Tashi, is still alive, I also want him there so I can feel his rich fur, receive his kisses, and relive the joyous times of reaching peaks atop the Continental Divide, which for me is as close as a mortal can get to heaven.

Losing oneself in such beauty combines well with losing the ego in meditation. Both are paths to that deeper level where we are free from loneliness and feel a part of something bigger. Regardless of whom we have around us, what many people fear most in dying is not only pain that we cannot manage but aloneness we cannot escape. There is an unavoidable sense of feeling solitary and separate in the process of dying. No one can die for us. No one can go with us on the journey. The peace that meditation brings, in both living and dying, comes from the sense of communion and harmony we have upon achieving it. As the young Dean Ornish, sick and depressed with a sense of failure (see Chapter 4) learned, meditation gives us an experience of belonging to something larger, beyond loneliness. For many, that something is God. "When a person has a sense of something greater than themselves, whatever it might be, it is very helpful when they are dying."[45]

GAINING A SENSE OF UNITY

The sense of unity that meditation brings was captured by pilgrims of the 12th Century who began the custom of walking labyrinths in the grand Gothic cathedrals of Europe. Instead of making pilgrimages to Jerusalem, which became too dangerous when the crusades swept across Europe, they went to such cathedrals as Chartres in France, where the Roman Church had installed labyrinth designs on the floor for people to walk in prayer and meditation. Labyrinths, whose spiral designs are found in nature (such as in the Golden Flower of ancient China), have been sacred symbols to humans for more than 4,000 years.[46] By following the one unicursal path to the labyrinth center, walkers would use it "to quiet the mind and find peace and illumination."[47] After a lapse of some 350 years, labyrinth walking is being revived in the United States. Rita and I walked the recently installed outdoor, stone labyrinth at the front of Grace Cathedral in San Francisco, a city that holds many memories for us of Liz, whom we took there as a little girl. We felt the quiet meeting of psyche and soul as we completed the 40-minute journey around the 11 circuits in and out of the labyrinth.

Mantras, the repeating of a given sound or word, are another way to go to our center of unity. In talks to doctors, nurses, psychologists, social workers, and hospice volunteers, Freeman points out the simplicity and power that mantra meditation has demonstrated for both the living and dying around the world for 5,000 years. He explains meditation this way:

> *Mantra* is a Sanskrit term that refers to a sacred text or phrase; it belongs to the traditions of every religious and spiritual family of humankind. It is within Christianity and Buddhism; it is within Hinduism, Judaism, and Islam. Its essential simplicity is at the centre of all human experience of prayer, of depth, of spirit. The word that you choose should naturally express your faith. For a Christian it would be a Christian word, for a Buddhist, a Buddhist word. The word that Father John recommended was the ancient Christian prayer word, *Maranatha*. Say it as four long single syllables of equal length, Ma-ra-na-tha. Sit down. Sit still. Close your eyes and silently, interiorly, begin to repeat your word from the beginning to the end.[48]

FEELING COMPLETE

But the degree of peace we achieve at death depends on more than just our meditation practice, prayers, and stories in the dying process. It is also a function of feeling complete about our lives in other ways as well. Completion involves more than the tangible matter of putting our affairs in order. It also requires our doing the intangible, emotional work of finishing what is incomplete in mourning our losses, which usually means our loved ones and our health.

We will go to great lengths to bring closure to the deaths of loved ones, and sometimes we have to go even further for bringing an end to our grief. After the long-unexplained explosion and crash of a TWA jumbo jet off Long Island in 1996, families waited months for bodies of their parents, children, and other relatives to be recovered from the sea. Finally, with 15 bodies still missing, their families gathered around 15 empty coffins for a funeral service in a Farmingdale, New York, cemetery. It was their way to give their dead closing rites. In another tribute of closure, a Houston man, whose wife and two daughters went down with the jumbo jet, rented a helicopter to fly over the site so he could drop roses into their ocean grave.

When we lose parts or use of our own body, when our health seems gone, we also need to mourn. John Callahan, at 21 an alcoholic who became quadriplegic after a night of drinking and a head-on crash at 90 miles an hour with a concrete entrance sign to a community college, slowly regained sobriety and sanity through an alcoholism support group. His last therapist asked him: "Did you ever mourn the loss of your twenty-one-year-old body?" Callahan had to say, "No, I didn't." By then he had a "hatred" for his body, now largely paralyzed, "because it's useless."[49] He acknowledged that "it's so difficult for me to get in touch with feelings," but probe them we must if we want to lighten our emotional load and move on in life.

OUR JOURNEY BACK

Shortly before the first anniversary of our daughter's death, I felt myself sliding into a depression over a replay of that loss. Contributing to that descent was the pain from my knee injury that wouldn't heal. My knees and legs had long served me well up and down mountains, on marathons, and on morning runs. Now I felt I was losing what I had taken for granted that my limbs would always do for me. I felt I was having to give up a way of life that had become a part of me. In the midst of this small sorrow, I also became slowly aware that I had more mourning to do over Liz's death.

Although my wife and I felt blessed that we had been given the chance to make peace with Liz and ourselves two years earlier when she was near death in the Intensive Care Unit (Chapter 4), the suddenness with which she finally died left me feeling incomplete. After her death, we took her ashes to the places she had requested they be distributed—to the Continental Divide, to the Caribbean, to Hawaii, each with a beauty she had loved. At the last place, in a quiet cove at Mauna Kea, we watched her dust return to the sand of the shallows and followed a gardenia Rita had placed at water's edge as it was slowly carried out to sea.

All of this helped fill the hole in my midsection from Liz's death, but I knew there was one more place I had to go for my completion: to the dark haunts of her life as an addict and to the scene of her death. At the time Liz died, it was enough to view and claim her body at the New York Medical Examiner's morgue, to talk with the pathologist—a kind, young woman not many years older than our dead daughter—who did her autopsy, to arrange for cremation, and to hold a memorial at the cathedral in her neighborhood so that Liz's friends could mourn her and say good-bye. I knew then I would have to come back to walk her path and see the place she died.

I kept postponing the return because of my own resistance to look more closely at the face of death and the darkness in Liz's soul and my own. I had the details of her death, but I did not want to see where she died. Two days after her death, I had received, totally unexpectedly, a long distance phone call from the young physician who tried to revive her in the emergency room at St. Luke's Hospital that late, final night. EMS had brought her in from the Upper West Side apartment building where she shared the room of a kindly old black man she had befriended. He was becoming increasingly feeble and gave Liz lodging in return for doing chores for him and walking and taking care of his aging dog. The ER physician said he called just to say he was sorry that there was nothing he could have done for her, that her massive internal bleeding had been beyond reversing. We talked a few minutes, and I thanked him for his efforts and kindness.

The same day I returned a call from the Fourth Precinct detective who had investigated her fall down 16 hard marble steps in the old upper West Side apartment building between Amsterdam and Broadway. He said she had been on the fifth floor with a man who was high on drugs and that when she left his room, she was unsteady and wobbling and tumbled down one flight of stairs. I already knew what to expect when months later I received the final toxicology and autopsy report from the Office of the Chief Medical Examiner of the City of New York: Her blood and brain were loaded with drugs, a mix of uppers and downers, from cocaine to heroin. With all the details complete and her ashes gone, I now knew I had to walk her path if I wanted to fill, at least in part, the aching hole in the pit of my stomach.

DESCENT INTO DARKNESS

Everything has its wonders,

Even darkness and silence, and I learn,

Whatever state I may be in,

Therein to be content.

—HELEN KELLER

When we finally made the trip back, I asked Donn Lowe to take me to the building where she died and to the streets that had become her home. Donn, a talented guitarist, band leader, and arranger, was Liz's best friend who tried to stay in touch with her as she made her descent into darkness. Rita and I became friends with him from long conversations over the telephone and meeting him at St. Luke's Hospital when Liz almost died two years earlier.

Rita, Donn, and I went to the apartment not too many blocks from the grand old Gothic Cathedral of St. John the Divine, where Liz had worked occasionally in the soup kitchen that fed the homeless in the area. It was not that much farther up Amsterdam Avenue to Columbia University, where I had gone to graduate school as a young man and walked the neighborhoods that I now was returning to on a much different mission.

The room Liz had shared with William "Satin" Hill was in a rundown old building that had once seen better days when the Amsterdam Avenue blocks near the cathedral were more affluent. Now it was a polyglot ghetto in which immigrants, welfare recipients, and sick and disabled persons on SSI (Supplemental Security Income) lived in one-room apartments crafted out of the once-spacious apartment buildings and nineteen-twentyish hotels. In

Liz's building, people occupying the dozen or so rooms on each floor shared three hallway bathrooms.

Satin was now in a nursing home, and his old apartment on the second floor was vacant. We knocked on the door of the adjoining room and had a long talk with José who had lived there for the last 25 years. He remembered Liz well. In accented English, he said he remembered "she was a sweet person and talked educated. With her, you wonder why she was here, living this sort of life. I saw her the day before she died. She said she was leaving. Satin was too sick for her to help him and he would have to go to the hospital."

We walked up to the fifth floor where Liz had been the night she died. Sixteen steps with one small landing in between separate the fifth and fourth floors. I wanted to see what Liz saw when she plunged to her death. Long dusty windows look out from the old marble stairway to a tiny playground out back separating her building and the next. A swing, a slide, a tree, and footprints in the small sandy area were the signs of life that were Liz's last earthly glimpse, conscious or unconscious as it was. It was a fitting final view. In her short life she kept seeing through her own dark pane the signs of a happier life on the other side, which she could never get back to.

But through it all, Liz had a bright side balancing the dark that never quite left her, even when she hit rock bottom. She managed to retain a capacity for hope and joy. She held on to a childlike quality, a kind of innocence, which she never lost even when her life began to unravel. Her watercolor art always had rainbow colors. In a trip with Rita and me to Hawaii, she had seen a spectacular double rainbow that she didn't forget. A priest she knew at the cathedral showed us a watercolor drawing she had inscribed to him shortly before her death. In the picture were high peaks and tiny figures of big-horn sheep she had seen on a whitewater rafting trip in the Salmon Mountains of Idaho. Above the peaks was a rainbow.

TRANSFORMING POWER

Even withered trees

give prosperity to the mountain.

—JAPANESE PROVERB

In the taxi to the airport after our visit, Rita and I talked about whether Liz's life had been a waste. From the outside it looked to many to be just that. Then I remembered the letter Donn Lowe wrote me after her death. "My memory of her is not of a bad wasted life but one of a friend that I loved deeply. She was kind and giving and had great sympathy, trying to cheer me up when I was out of work, even though she had her own pain. I understand now the pain of addiction. She told me many times not to give up on her, and I never did. She taught me how to love and give to others. She gave me confidence and strength. She changed my life." Later, I told Donn of how I was changed by Liz's life: she taught me more patience and humility, and the wisdom of letting go.

The theme of this book has been how pain is transmuted into something positive, how it can be used to change us and others for the better. In the opening chapters I spoke of the kind of alchemy worked by those in pain, sickness, and impairment who have succeeded in converting dross into gold. This is how the sick stay well.

For those who think they will never succeed in using their pain in such a way, there is an image of God as the great alchemist who has the genius to take the consequences of even the worst in us, among us, and around us and turn it into something good and lasting. Accordingly, God wastes nothing. He only transforms: weakness into strength, darkness into light, pain into peace, sickness into health.

The transformation that is ours to make is expanding our awareness to see this as our destiny, so that we know at the deepest level of our health and self that "all is or will be well."[50]

Chapter One—BEING WELL INSIDE OURSELVES

1. Kawaga–Singer, 1993.
2. *Healthy People 2000,* 1991.
3. Myers, 1992, p. 24.
4. Kutner, 1994; Kaplan, & Camacho, 1983; Myers, 1992.
5. Idler, & Kasl, 1991, p. S55.
6. Patrick, & Erickson, 1993; Kaplan, 1995; Vaillant, 1977; Kutner, 1994; Barsky, Cleary, & Klerman, 1992.
7. Idler, 1995. It took me a long time to discover my nonphysical health. The work of Ellen Idler made me realize how many others have found theirs.
8. Dossey, 1984. I wasn't ready to believe there was a health beyond the physical when Larry Dossey first wrote of it. By the time I re-read *Beyond Illness* I knew from living it that there is a different kind of health.
9. Topf, with Bennett, 1995, p. 18.
10. Ibid., p. 14.
11. Kawaga–Singer, 1993, p. 295.
12. Idler, & Angel, 1990.
13. Scheier, & Carver, 1985; Roush, 1997; Sternberg, 1997. Although Sternberg's evidence is on emotions affecting physiological processes, belief (thoughts, attitudes, appraisal) precede most emotions, as established by numerous empirical studies.
14. Justice, 1988; Benson, & Epstein, 1975; Benson, 1995; Benson, & Friedman, 1996; Benson, 1996. Dr. Herbert Benson was a mainstream medicine pioneer in demonstrating through the placebo effect that what we believe affects what our bodily systems do.
15. Blau, 1985, p. 344.
16. Seligman, 1991.
17. Lovallo, 1997.
18. Myers, 1992, p. 24. It seems appropriate that the author of *Pursuit of Happiness* should be at Hope College. At age 49, as he was writing

this well-documented book, he knew he was going deaf. "I find my hearing declining on a trajectory directly toward my 82-year-old mother's utter deafness." Wearing a hearing aid and using amplification devices for TV and telephone, Myers is confident that his core well-being will remain with him.

19. Justice, 1988; Phillips, & Smith, 1990; Phillips, & King, 1988.
20. Allan, & Scheidt, 1996.
21. Johns Hopkins Medical Letter: Health after 50, July 1997.
22. Idler, & Kasl, 1991, p. S55.
23. Rinpoche, 1992.
24. Cannon, 1942.
25. Kaplan, 1995, p. 10. Kaplan is citing statistics from the RAND Health Insurance Study.
26. Taylor, 1995, p. 450.
27. Kaplan, 1995, p. 10.
28. Shuman, 1996, p. 8.
29. Murphy, 1987, p. 87.
30. Kaplan, Barell, & Lusky, 1988, p. S114.
31. Shuman, 1996, p. 8.
32. Frank, 1991; Frank, 1995.
33. Bolen, 1996, p. 192.
34. Hahn, 1995; Lock, 1980; Hahn, 1984.
35. Kawaga-Singer, 1993, p. 295; Parsons, 1958.
36. Kawaga-Singer, 1993, p. 295.
37. Murphy, Scheer, Murphy, & Mack, 1988, p. 237.
38. Gomes, 1996, p. 215.
39. Myers, 1992.
40. Hahn, 1995; Kutner, 1994.
41. As director and principal investigator of this pilot project, I did in-depth, 90-minute psychological interviews with 13 of the women after our controlled clinical trial had ended. In this study, we compared the effects of imagery and support versus standard care on immune function, mood state, ways of coping, meaning, and coherence in 47 women treated for breast cancer (see Richardson et al., 1997). Those participating in the qualitative interviews were chosen on the basis of their availability to be interviewed in their home or workplace or my office. Delores formerly worked at M.D.

Anderson and was familiar with the Texas Medical Center, so she chose to come to the School of Public Health, across the street from Anderson, to be interviewed.

42. Delores. Interview with author, September 17, 1996.
43. Mount, 1996a, p. 8.
44. World Health Organization, 1947.
45. *Healthy People: 2000,* 1991.
46. Patrick, & Erickson, 1993; Kaplan, 1995.
47. Benson, 1996, pp. 49–59; Vaillant, 1977, p. 13.
48. Justice, 1988.
49. Dossey, 1984, p.35.
50. Ibid., p. 36.
51. Ibid.
52. Ibid., p. 37.
53. Ibid.
54. Barsky, Cleary, & Klerman, 1992; Kaplan, Barell, & Lusky, 1988.
55. Verbrugge, & Balaban, 1989, p. S128.
56. Koenig, 1995.
57. Nelson, 1996.
58. Miller, 1991.
59. Ibid.
60. Ibid.
61. Riley, Ahern, & Follick, 1988; Benson, 1996, p. 60.
62. Phillips, Ruth, & Wagner, 1993.
63. Benson, 1996, p. 318; Riley, Ahern, & Follick, 1988.
64. Styron, 1990.
65. Koenig, 1995.
66. Antonovsky, 1987, p. 14; See also, Fries, & Crapo, 1981.
67. *Alternative Medicine: Expanding Medical Horizons,* 1992, p. ix; *Healthy People 2000,* 1991.
68. *Alternative Medicine,* 1992, p. ix.
69. Koenig, 1995.
70. Idler, & Kasl, 1992.
71. Frank, 1991, p. 130.
72. Frank, 1991, p. 7.
73. Ibid.

Chapter Two—SHIFTING OUR IDENTITY

1. Dienstfrey, 1992, p. 34; Bensen, 1996; Chopra, 1991.
2. Kawaga-Singer, 1993.
3. Benson, 1995; Ferguson, 1996, p. 5; James, & James, 1991.
4. Dienstfrey, 1992; Bensen, 1996; Chopra, 1991.
5. Stapp, 1993, p. 213.
6. Watts, 1996.
7. Lawlis, 1996a; Hagelin, 1983.
8. Chopra, 1991, p. 313.
9. Lawlis, 1996a, p. 5.
10. Wordsworth, 1807.
11. Harman, 1997, p. 15.
12. Ibid., p. 16.
13. As quoted by Walsh and Walsh, 1989, p. 797.
14. Ephron, 1987, as quoted in Dossey, 1991, p. 139.
15. Berendt, 1987, p. 171.
16. Pert, as quoted in an interview by Bonnie Horrigan, 1995, p. 76.
17. Buechner, 1996, p. 106.
18. Ibid., p. 107.
19. Ibid.
20. Cohen, & Mount, 1992, p. 41.
21. Mount, 1993.
22. For more on being well inside the self, see Byock, 1997.
23. Maer, Leventhal, & Johnson, 1992.
24. Janoff-Bulman, & Timko, 1987.
25. Veatch, 1997.
26. Kaplan, Barell, & Lusky, 1988.
27. Ibid., p. S115.
28. Ibid., p. S118.
29. Parsons, 1958.
30. Kasl, & Cobb, 1966.
31. Kawaga-Singer, 1993, p. 295.
32. Murphy, Sheer, Murphy, & Mack, 1988, p. 238.
33. Frank, 1995, p. 9.
34. Nucho, 1988.
35. Broyard, 1992, p. 45.

36. Brody, 1987.
37. Clearman, 1996. The trauma of losing facial identity has been dealt with in various ways throughout history. In the early 19th century the beautiful wife of Irish poet Thomas Moore didn't give up her will to live because of disfigurement from smallpox but resolved to close herself off to her husband and the world so no one would see her. It was only after Moore found the right words for a poem he dedicated to his wife and sung to her in her darkened room that she got out of bed, opened the shutters, and let the light of a dawning day pour into the room and onto her disfigured face. The poem ends with the words, "Let thy loveliness fade as it will/and round the dear ruin each wish of my heart/Would entwine itself verdantly still." I heard Rev. David Tetrault sing the words of Moore's poem in a sermon he gave June 29, 1997, during the 300th anniversary celebration of Grace Episcopal Church in Yorktown, Virginia.
38. Antonovsky, 1987.
39. Damasio, Grabowski, Frank, Galabarda, & Damasio, 1994, p. 1102.
40. Ibid.
41. Benson, 1996, p. 81.
42. Melzack, 1992, p. 314; Gazzanica, 1988.
43. Sachs, 1990.
44. Sachs, 1991, p. 368.
45. Eliot, 1963, p. 199.
46. Sachs, 1987, p. 39.
47. Ibid.
48. Fordyce, 1988; Fordyce, Brockway, Bergman, & Spengler, 1986.
49. Damasio, 1994, p. 54.
50. Sachs, 1991, p. 369.
51. Benner, & Wrubel, 1989.
52. Rein, Atkinson, & McCraty, 1995.
53. Mathew, 1995.

Chapter Three—IMPROVING AS A PERSON

1. Taylor, 1989; Hirshberg, & Barasch, 1995; Wholey, 1992.
2. Janoff-Bulman, & Timko, 1987.

3. Taylor, 1989; Myers, 1992; Frank, 1991.
4. Lerner, 1990, p. 191.
5. Rowland, 1997.
6. Goodare, 1997, p. 36.
7. Goethals, & Strauss, 1991, p. 238.
8. See Evelyn Fox Keller's biography of McClintock, 1983.
9. Ibid., p. 200.
10. Fryback, 1993.
11. Carter, 1991, p. 354.
12. Ibid.
13. Ibid., p. 358.
14. Buchholz, & Buchholz, 1997, p. 6.
15. Hirshberg, & Barasch, 1995, pp. 181–184.
16. Ibid., p. 183.
17. Ibid., p. 184.
18. Turnbull, Patterson, Behr, Murphy, Marquis, & Blue-Banning, 1993.
19. Newman, 1986, p. 20.
20. Fryback, 1993, p. 157.
21. Henrich, & Kriegel, 1961, p. 19.
22. Anna. Interview with author, August 29, 1996.
23. Dossey, L., 1995, p. 6.
24. Ibid.
25. Ibid, p. 8.
26. Buckman, 1992, pp. 9–14.
27. Ibid, p. 12.
28. Most disabilities do not come from injuries but from diseases, such as those affecting muscles, bones or tissue, the circulatory system, respiration, the nervous system, glands or the immune system. Insurance companies are starting to promote rehabilitation programs to help disabled people to return to work. An example was a five-day camping and canoeing trip in the Everglades wilderness sponsored by Hartford Life Insurance Company. On the trip, "there was no high-tech therapy. Rather, like Outward Bound excursions so popular with young people, its purpose was to help participants discover unsuspected reserves of strength for overcoming adversity.

It was also a way for Hartford to showcase its new emphasis on rehabilitation." (Treaster, 1997, C4).

29. Affleck, & Tennen, 1993, p. 138.
30. Meyer, 1993, p. 84.
31. Eliot, & Breo, 1984, p. 1.
32. Ibid., p. 7.
33. Ibid.
34. Affleck, & Tennen, 1993, p. 139.
35. Lawlis, 1996b.
36. Lawlis, 1996a, p. 222.
37. Ibid., p. 225.
38. Affleck, & Tennen, 1993, p. 138.
39. Dana. Interview with author, July 19, 1996.
40. Walsh, & Walsh, 1989, p. 793.
41. Lawlis, 1996b, p. 64.
42. Buber, 1987; Erikson, 1963.
43. Shakespeare, 1955c, p. 52.
44. Cohen, 1993. Dr. Peter Morgan, another of the physicians in the remarkable teaching video *On the Edge of Being* was diagnosed with a metastatic sarcoma of the right leg at age 29 just as he had accepted an ontology fellowship after finishing his residency. He used his experience as a patient to teach fellow physicians to treat the whole person and not just the physical part. In a diary Morgan kept after his diagnosis, he wrote this challenge to his tumor: "You won't even touch my daily spirit of life and my immortal soul" *(USA Today,* June 27, 1997, p. 3D). A public broadcasting system TV documentary by Ruth Yorkin Drazen was made based on Morgan's diary, testifying that "within the chaos of illness, he found purpose and peace."
45. Affleck, & Tennen, 1993, p. 139.
46. Ibid. See a study by Affleck, Tennen, & Rowe, 1990.
47. Affleck, & Tennen, 1993, p. 139.
48. Taylor, Kemeny, Reed, & Aspinwall, 1991.
49. Taylor, 1989.
50. Breznitz, 1983.
51. Janoff-Bulman, & Timko, 1987, p. 155.

52. James, & James, 1991, p. 216.
53. Larson, 1995.
54. Garraty, & Gay, 1987.
55. Idler, 1995.
56. Frank, 1991, p. 121.
57. Taylor, 1995, p. 442.
58. Frank, 1991, p. 135.
59. Suchman, & Matthews, 1988, p. 126.
60. Ibid.
61. Ibid.
62. Ibid.
63. Buchholz, & Buchholz, 1997.
64. Katie. Interview with author, September 5, 1996.
65. Okun, Stock, Haring, & Witter, 1984, p. 114.
66. Frankl, 1996, p. 20.
67. Smith, 1986.
68. McEntyre, 1995, p. 95.
69. Feifel, 1990, p. 541.
70. Feifel, 1969, p. 294.
71. McEntyre, 1995, p. 95.
72. Antonovsky, 1987, p. 2; See also, Fries, & Crapo, 1981, p. 14.
73. Antonovsky, 1979; Antonovsky, 1987.
74. Antonovsky, 1987, p. 16.
75. Vaillant, 1977; Vaillant, & Vaillant, 1990.
76. Vaillant, 1977, p. 16.
77. Vaillant, 1977; Vaillant, 1990.
78. Merchant, 1991, p. 7.
79. Myers, 1992, p. 48.
80. Ibid.
81. Ibid.
82. Taylor, Lichtman, & Wood, 1984; Taylor, & Aspinwall, 1990; Taylor, 1995.
83. Taylor, 1995, p. 450.
84. Tempellar, De Haes, De Ruiter, Bakker, Van Den Heuvel, & Van Nieuwenhuijzen, 1989; Taylor, et al., 1991, p. 240.
85. Druss, & Douglas, 1988.
86. Trillin, 1981.

87. Ibid., p. 701.
88. Lilly. Interview with author, August 7, 1996.

Chapter Four—DISCOVERING A NEW KIND OF HEALTH

1. Fryback, 1993.
2. Block, 1997, p. 6.
3. Cassell, 1982.
4. Freud, 1955, p. 28.
5. Gomes, 1996, p. 221.
6. Kliever, 1989, p. xi.
7. Cowart, 1996.
8. Ibid.
9. Cassell, 1982, p. 644.
10. Ornish, 1990.
11. Gould, Ornish, Scherwitz, Brown, Edens, Hess, Mullani, Bolomey, Dobbs, & Armstrong, 1995; Ornish, 1993.
12. Horrigan, 1995a, p. 91.
13. Ornish, 1990, p. 109.
14. Ornish, 1990, p. 110.
15. Ornish, 1997.
16. Gomes, 1996, p. 236.
17. Ibid., p. 243.
18. Spiegel, 1993.
19. Thoreau, 1960, p. 39.
20. Ibid.
21. As quoted by Dossey, 1984, p. 26.
22. Spiegel, Bloom, Kraemer, & Gottheil, 1989.
23. Spiegel, 1993, p. 257.
24. Ibid.
25. Benson, 1996, p. 157.
26. Delbruck, 1971, p. 55. The code, the guiding intelligence of the DNA base pairing and sequencing, is invisible in the sense spirit or soul is and in the sense of whatever the motive force is that guides development from fertilized egg to adult organism. Most biological scientists who work on the molecular level deny there is any

motive force and hold that mechanical laws can explain the "intelligent" development from egg to maturity. This position has not been confirmed by empirical evidence.

27. Sheldrake, 1985.
28. Pert interview by Horrigan, 1995b, p. 75.
29. Broyard, 1992, p. 40.
30. James, & James, 1991, p. 21.
31. Ibid.
32. As quoted in Wakefield, 1996, p. 25.
33. Shakespeare, 1955b, p. 775.
34. Jung, as quoted in Jaffe, 1965.
35. Buber, 1969, P. 49.
36. Kass, 1988a, p. 2.
37. Kass, 1988b, pp. 4–5.
38. As quoted in Moore, 1989, p. 26.
39. Wolf, as quoted in an interview with Johnson, 1997.
40. Ibid.
41. Ibid., p. 4.
42. Mora, 1963. Another way to think about conatus and our molecular "strivings" is to shift our basic ontological assumption about living organisms. Rather than seeing them, as modern science does, as inorganic matter organized by the mechanical motions of molecules, a different assumption would be that all sentient beings, all organisms, consist of living matter infused by spirit or consciousness. For more on this, see Harman, 1997.
43. Antonovsky, 1992.
44. Post-White, 1993.
45. Antonovsky, 1987, p. 17.
46. Ibid., pp. 17–18.
47. Antonovsky, 1987.
48. Bulman & Wortman, 1977; Turnbull, Patterson, Behr, Murphy, Marquis, & Blue-Banning, 1993; Myers, 1992.
49. Myers, 1992, p. 50.
50. Lilly. Interview with author, August 7, 1996.
51. Wakefield, 1996.
52. Myers, 1992, p. 49.
53. Remen, 1996, pp. 193–194.

54. Ibid.
55. Conversation with author, February 1, 1997. Commonweal Conference on New Directions in Health and Healing, Bolinas, California.
56. Lusseyran, 1959.
57. Mishra, 1962.
58. Wheeler, 1977.
59. McEntyre, 1995, p. 88.
60. Ibid., p. 87.
61. Dillard, 1988, pp. 14–15.
62. *Alternative Medicine: Expanding Medical Horizons.* A Report to the National Institutes of Health. Washington, DC: Government Printing Office, 1994, p. 4.
63. Lerner, 1994.
64. Remen, 1996, p. xxiv.
65. Ibid.
66. Ibid., p. xxv.

Chapter Five—APPRECIATING WHAT IS

1. Sheed, 1989, p. 71.
2. Price, 1994; Williams, 1989; Frank, 1991; Styron, 1990.
3. Kabat-Zinn, 1990.
4. See Ellen Langer's 1989 book, *Mindfulness,* for early evidence on the power that this way of being aware in life can have on physical and psychological well-being.
5. Kabat-Zinn, 1990, p. 5.
6. As quoted in an interview by Avrel Seale, 1997, p. 28. Prigogine disputes Einstein's view that "everything is determined. He thought," Prigogine says, "we are automata without knowing we are automata." Prigogine holds a more "optimistic view" of us and the universe and believes that "creativity is a very basic experience of human experience" and novelty is a characteristic of nature.
7. Ibid.
8. Cousins, 1989, pp. 146–147.
9. McCraty, Atkinson, Tiller, Rein, & Watkins, 1995; *BrainMind Bulletin,* November 1995, p. 1.

10. Ibid.
11. McCraty, Atkinson, Tiller, Rein, & Watkins, 1995, p. 1092.
12. McCraty, Atkinson, & Tiller, 1995, p. 267.
13. Justice, 1988.
14. Zajonc, 1985.
15. Mayne, 1997.
16. Blum, 1997. Dr. Blum, an associate professor of family medicine at Baylor College of Medicine, sketches many of his patients (with their permission) as a way to get inside their lives and know them better. His drawings have been published in *JAMA* and other medical journals.
17. Rysavy, as quoted by Locke, 1997, pp. 1D, 14–16D.
18. Ibid., p. 14D.
19. Gallagher, 1989, Introduction, p. xxii.
20. Carver, 1989, p. 118.
21. Ibid., p. 117.
22. Gallagher, Introduction, 1989, p. xxvii.
23. Carver, 1989, p. 122.
24. Dimsdale, 1974.
25. A book, *Song of Survival,* by Helen Colijn, tells of the "etherial" effects the women created with their chorus and music. Their spirit is captured in a 1997 movie, "Paradise Lost," based on the book, in which Glenn Close plays a leading role.
26. Stronck, as quoted by Parks, 1997.
27. Ibid.
28. Klein, 1988, p. 308.
29. Wordsworth, 1798, pp. 114–115.
30. Klein, 1988, p. 308.
31. Stevens, 1993, p. B5.
32. Dorothy. Interview with author, July 22, 1996.
33. Thorne, 1993.
34. Klein, 1988, p. 308.
35. Buechner, 1992, p. 113.
36. Gordon, 1993.
37. Friedman, Powell, Thoresen, Ulmer, Price, Gill, Thompson, Rabin, Brown, Breall, et al., 1987.
38. Thoresen, 1989.

39. Singer, 1996, p. 2.
40. Moore, 1996, p. 103.
41. Singer, 1996, p.2.
42. Hillman, 1993.
43. Ellis, 1923, p. 328.
44. Moyers, 1982.
45. Heisenberg, 1974, p. 183.
46. Watson, 1968, pp. 131, 134.
47. Zwinger, & Willard, 1972, pp. 3–4.
48. Augros, & Stanciu, 1984.
49. Dannen, & Dannen, 1981, pp. 7–8.
50. Cushman, Jones, with Knopf, 1993, p. 199.
51. Raver, 1994, p. C1.
52. Ibid.
53. Messervy, 1995, p. 11.
54. Rumi, as quoted in Messervy, 1995, p. 13.
55. Messervy, 1995, p. 19.
56. Miller, 1995, p. 180.
57. Thomas, 1992.
58. Shepherd, 1994.
59. Olman, 1995.
60. Mary. Interview with author, August 7, 1996.
61. Ibid.

Chapter Six—MAKING OUR PAIN SING

1. Morris, 1991.
2. Wedemeyer, 1996, p. 22.
3. Ibid.
4. Bauby, 1997; see also Mallon, 1997.
5. Bauby, 1997, p. 5, p. 36.
6. Morris, 1995, p. 21.
7. Gazzaniga, 1988.
8. Hanson, 1990; Caudill, 1995.
9. Morris, 1995, p. 18.
10. House, Landis, & Umberson, 1988; Topf, with Bennett, 1995.

11. Remen, 1988, p. 6.
12. Ibid., p. 8.
13. Ibid.
14. Morris, 1991, p. 197.
15. Cousins, 1990.
16. Alternative Medicine: Expanding Medical Horizons, 1994, pp 98–99.
17. Baker, 1981, p. 408.
18. Coffee, as quoted in Hirshberg, & Barasch, 1995, p. 183. See also Blaise Pascal's "Prayer to ask God for the good use of sickness," (Prière pour demander á dieu le bon usage des maladies), in Lafuma, 1963, pp. 363–364.
19. Rimer, 1995, p. A8.
20. Anderson, & Warnock, 1967, p. III: 450.
21. Keats, in Anderson, & Warnock, 1967, p. III: 452.
22. Anderson, & Warnock, 1967, p. III: 450.
23. Keats, as quoted in Cheyne, 1983, p. 28.
24. Anderson, & Warnock, 1967, p. III: 459.
25. Robertson. Personal communication, April 26, 1996.
26. Dorothy. Interview with author, July 22, 1996.
27. Ellen. Interview with author, July 22, 1996.
28. Lilly. Interview with author, August 7, 1996.
29. Matlin, 1991, as presented in Friend, & the Editors of Life, p. 95.
30. Deanna. Interview with author, August 20, 1996.
31. Sandy. Interview with author, July 23, 1996.

Chapter Seven—LIVING WITH PURPOSE

1. McHugh, 1997, p. 26. Another neuroscientist, Nobelist Roger Sperry and 1989 winner of the National Medal of Science, also had PLS (primary lateral sclerosis) and remarkably continued his work. He became a vocal spokesman for "top-down" theories on how mind and consciousness, particularly values and ideas, have strong neural and physiological effect on the brain and body. I am aware that both Butters and Sperry had a rich inner life that they

drew on to go beyond their physical disability. Many of us are not that cerebral. Some who have lived their lives working more with their hands and requiring great physical stamina may wish to die when their bodies fail them.

Such was the case with the father of Pat Morrison of the *Los Angeles Times.* She gave a moving account on public radio (March 11, 1997) of her father's decline from a form of Lou Gehrig's disease and her determination to assist him in his wish to die. Her father, Gene, had been a lineman on high power lines for many years and loved work and physical activity so much, his fellow workers called him, "Gene, Gene, the Machine." He was a runner and a man in perpetual motion. When his disease robbed him of his strength, he made it plain he didn't want to wait for death to come. His daughter carefully researched what pills and dosage were necessary to induce death in Gene, who chose a particular flavored milkshake for the pills to be mixed in. On the day he and his family chose for his death, he made their assistance unnecessary. He succeeded in willing himself to death.

2. Ibid., p. 25.
3. Ibid., p. 26.
4. Ibid.
5. Frankl, 1963, p. 20.
6. Gazzaniga, 1988, p. 20.
7. Morris, 1991, p. 194.
8. Fordyce, 1988, p. 282.
9. Seligman, 1989, p. 94; Seligman, 1988.
10. Jung, 1931/1962, p. 91. The Golden Flower resembles labyrinths and mandalas in design. See Chapter 10.
11. Myers, 1992, p. 189; Csikszentimihaly, 1990.
12. Affleck, & Tennen, 1993, p. 137.
13. Ibid.
14. Affleck, & Tennen, 1991; Affleck, & Tennen, 1993, p. 138.
15. Myers, 1992.
16. Friedman, Powell, Thoresen, Ulmer, Price, Gill, Thompson, Rabin, Brown, Breall, et al., 1987; Dienstfrey, 1992, p. 34; Ornish, 1995, p. 84; Bracke, & Thoresen, 1996.
17. Thoresen, 1989.

18. Ibid.
19. Scherwitz, McKelvain, Laman, Patterson, Dutton, Yusim, Lester, Kraft, Rochelle, & Leachman, 1983.
20. Bellah, Madsen, Sullivan, Swidler, & Tipton, 1985.
21. Ornish, 1993.
22. Thoresen, 1989.
23. Dossey, 1995, pp. 6–7.
24. Ibid., p. 7.
25. Ayto, 1990, p. 141.
26. Shakespeare, 1955a, p. 613.
27. Tillich, 1952, p. 3.
28. Ibid.
29. Ibid., pp. 4–5.
30. Jung, as quoted in Jaffe, 1965, p. 4.
31. L'Engle, 1980, p. 62.
32. Ibid.
33. Ibid., p. 63.
34. Krauss, & Goldfischer, 1990, p. xiv.
35. Ibid.
36. Ibid., p. 12.
37. Ibid., p. 13.
38. Remen, 1988, p. 5.
39. Hammond, 1996.
40. Robertson, 1990; Miller, 1984.
41. Miller, 1984, p. 77.
42. Robertson, 1990, p. 13.
43. Miller, 1984, p. 77.
44. Ibid.
45. Miller, 1984, p. 98.
46. Feuerstein, Labbé, & Kuczmierczyk, 1986.
47. Lawlis, 1996a, p. 193.
48. Kosambi, 1967.
49. Kübler-Ross, 1970; Justice, 1988.
50. Phillips, & King, 1988.
51. Ibid., p. 728.
52. Ibid., p. 732.
53. Ibid.

54. Peete, 1990, p. 2. Dr. Peete went on to become an associate clinical professor of medicine and lecturer in the history of medicine at the University of Kansas School of Medicine and was an early champion of mind body health. He was the author of *The Psychosomatic Genesis of Coronary Artery Disease* (Springfield, IL: Charles C Thomas, 1955).
55. Adolphe, 1996.
56. Monsaingeon, 1988, p. 117.
57. Ibid., p. 10.
58. Ibid., p. 119.

Chapter Eight—FINDING FAITH

1. Brooks, 1989, p. 104.
2. Brooks, 1989.
3. Pascal, 1966.
4. St. George, & McNamara, 1984, p. 351.
5. See Kant in Palmer, 1988, pp. 206–222.
6. Benson, 1996.
7. Myers, 1992.
8. Persinger, 1987. More recently, other researchers reported at the 1997 conference of the Society for Neuroscience on finding a "God module" in the temporal lobe of the brain.
9. Ibid., p. 14.
10. Fant, & Ashley, 1964, p. 80.
11. Dobyzhansky, 1967.
12. Montagu, 1942.
13. Rousseau, as quoted in Garraty, & Gay, 1987, p. 720.
14. Cassell, 1982, p. 643.
15. Hay, 1982, p. 193; Hardy, 1975.
16. As quoted in Mitchell, & Williams, 1996, p. 40.
17. Idler, 1995.
18. Mark 9:24.
19. As quoted in Lerner, 1990, p. 15.
20. Wolf, as quoted by Johnson, 1997.

21. Sheldrake, 1994, p. 6.
22. Ibid.
23. Ibid., p. 7.
24. Ibid., p. 7.
25. Ibid., p. 7.
26. Delores. Interview with author, September 17, 1996.
27. Dossey, 1996, p. 3.
28. Ibid.
29. Ibid.
30. Ibid.
31. Dossey, 1994.
32. Dossey, 1996, p. 3.
33. Benor, 1990; Benor, 1993; Dossey, 1993.
34. Dossey, 1994.
35. Marwick, 1995.
36. Ibid., p. 1562.
37. Kark, Shemi, Friedlander, Martin, Manor, & Blondheim, 1996.
38. Koenig, Cohen, George, Hays, Larson, & Blazer, 1997.
39. As reported by Schlitz, & Lewis, 1996.
40. Larson, & Witham, 1997; Angier, 1997.
41. Mellen, 1996.
32. Henneman, 1996, p. 2.
43. Ibid.
44. Affleck, & Tennen, 1993; Taylor, 1989.
45. Jacquelyn. Interview with author, August 7, 1996.
46. Lilly. Interview with author, August 7, 1996.
47. Gomes, 1996, p. 219.
48. Ibid., p. 222.
49. Polanyi, 1962.
50. Booth, 1990.
51. Hebrews 11:1, 1984, p. 1335.
52. Frankl, 1963.
53. May, 1988.
54. Ellison, & Smith, 1991.
55. Schmidt, 1993.
56. Williams, 1989.
57. Mathew, 1995.

Chapter Nine—BOUNCING BACK: AGAIN AND AGAIN

1. Fine, 1991.
2. Medalie, & Goldbourt, 1976.
3. Reifman, 1995, p. 124.
4. Suchman, & Matthews, 1988, p. 126.
5. Ibid., p. 127.
6. Ibid.
7. Lerner, 1994.
8. Lynch, 1977.
9. Field et al., 1986.
10. Field, 1993.
11. Reynolds, & Kaplan, 1990; Williams, Barefoot, Califf, Haney, Saunders, Pryor, Hlatky, Siegler, & Mark, 1992; Goodwin, Hunt, Key, & Samet, 1987.
12. Ditto, Druley, Moore, Danks, & Smucker, 1996.
13. Mount, 1996a, p. 8.
14. Justice, 1988.
15. Sorokin, 1964. Sorokin's survey research also discovered a number of "altruistic atheists," who practiced all the tenets of the Golden Rule outside any belief in God or affiliation with a religion. See also Matter, 1974.
16. Ornish, 1990; Lerner, 1994; Siegel, 1986.
17. Mayer, 1989, p. 78.
18. Lawlor, 1996, p. 20.
19. Messereni, 1984; Friedmann, Katcher, Thomas, Lynch, & Messent, 1983; Friedmann, Katcher, Lynch, & Thomas, 1980; Kalfon, 1991.
20. Langer, & Rodin, 1976.
21. Topping, 1997, p. 9F. A poem by Theodore Stephanides accompanied Topping's piece on Charlie in the *Houston Chronicle*. It's called "Epitaph for a Parrot":

> For thirty years he talked
> in feathered pride.
> For thirty years he talked
> before he died.
> You say that parrots do not
> really know

> The meaning of the words they use?
> Just so.
> I grant you that you might
> be right—but then
> Do Men?

22. Brody, 1996b, p. B9.
23. Ibid.
24. Goleman, 1996, p. A1.
25. Kolata, 1996, p. A1.
26. Brody, 1996a, p. B9.
27. Azar, 1996, p. 27.
28. Violet's insatiable curiosity about the world reminds me of Saul Bellow's advice to approach life with fresh eyes, as a newcomer on earth would. Bellow, 81, a Nobel laureate in literature, acts as if "I've never seen the world before. Now I was seeing it, and it's a beautiful, marvelous gift. Enchanting reality!" (See Gussow, 1997, p B1).
29. Idler, 1993.
30. Ibid., p. 220.
31. Petit, 1996.
32. Tye, 1977; Rosenberg, 1997.
33. Justice, 1988; Antoni, et al., 1991.
34. Lerner, 1994, p. 5.
35. LeShan, 1994, p. 219.
36. Ibid., p. 220.
37. Druss, & Douglas, 1988.
38. Ibid., p. 164.
39. Mairs, as quoted in Fine, 1991, p. 496.
40. Ibid.
41. Massimini, as cited by Csikszentmihalyi in Wholey, 1992, p. 148–151.
42. Csikszentmihalyi, as quoted in Wholey, 1992, p. 150.
43. Ibid.
44. Lawlor, 1996, p. 20.
45. Ibid.
46. Fannie Tapper. Interviews with the author, February 5, 1997 and March 13, 1997.
47. *Methodist Times:* Medical Staff, 1995.

48. Kobasa, 1979.
49. Buchholz, & Buchholz, 1997, p. 6.
50. Pennebaker, 1990.
51. Pennebaker, 1995.
52. Ibid., p. 17.
53. Mishlove, 1989.
54. Jenkins, 1989.
55. Claypool, 1992.
56. Isaiah 40:11.

Chapter Ten—DYING WELL

1. Freeman, 1996, p. 29.
2. Meyer, 1991.
3. Donnelley, 1982.
4. Hope, 1987.
5. LeShan, 1994, p. 163.
6. Ibid., p. 164.
7. Ibid.
8. Ibid., p. 165.
9. Ibid., p. 169.
10. Byock, 1997, p. xiv.
11. Remen, 1997.
12. *Corinthians 12:26.*
13. Ornish, as quoted in Remen, 1996, Foreword.
14. Sharkey, 1982.
15. Sharkey, 1982, p. 9.
16. Byock, 1997.
17. Ibid., p. 31.
18. Dossey, 1994.
19. Meyer, 1991, p. 84.
20. Nuland, 1994, p. 265.
21. Ibid., p. 266.
22. Ibid., p. 268.
23. Mattlin, 1996, p. 4C.
24. Ibid.

25. Byock, 1997, p. 36.
26. Remen, 1996, p. xxix.
27. Cohen, & Mount, 1992, p. 41.
28. Ibid.
29. Ibid.
30. Lerner, 1994.
31. Ibid., p. 492.
32. Ibid.
33. Nuland, 1994, p. 265.
34. Ibid.
35. Ibid.
36. Mount, 1996a, p. 7.
37. See Freeman, 1996, p. 13. Also see Main, 1981.
38. Freeman, 1994, p. 31.
39. Mount, 1996b.
40. Freeman, 1996, pp. 13–14.
41. Jung, 1965, p. 295.
42. Adler, 1975.
43. Jaffe, 1979.
44. *I Corinthians 15*:48–49, 1987; Jung, as quoted in Jaffe, 1979, p. 217.
45. Levine, 1990, as quoted in Lerner, 1994, p. 497.
46. Artress, 1995.
47. Artress, 1995, p. 1.
48. Freeman, 1996, p. 18.
49. Wholey, 1992, p. 19.
50. Myers, 1992, p. 24

REFERENCES

———————————————————✳———————————————————

Adler, G. (1975, July 14). Interview. British Broadcasting Company.

Adolphe, B. (1996). *What to Listen for in the World*. New York: Proscenium.

Affleck, G., Tennen, H., & Rowe, J. (1990). Mothers, fathers, and the crisis of newborn intensive care. *Infant Mental Health Journal, 11*, 12–25.

Affleck, G., & Tennen, H. (1991). Appraisal and coping predictors of mothers and child outcomes after newborn intensive care. *Journal of Social and Clinical Psychology, 10*, 424–447.

Affleck, G., & Tennen, H. (1993). Cognitive adaptation to adversity: Insights from parents of medically fragile infants. In A.P. Turnbull, et al., (Eds.), *Cognitive Coping, Families, and Disability* (pp. 135–150). Baltimore: Paul H. Brookes.

Allan, R., & Scheidt, S. (Eds.). (1996). *Heart & Mind: The Practice of Cardiac Psychology*. Washington, DC: American Psychological Association.

Alternative Medicine: Expanding Medical Horizons. (1994). A Report to the National Institutes of Health on Alternative Medical Systems and Practices in the United States. Washington, DC: Government Printing Office.

Anderson, G.K., & Warnock, R. (1967). *The World in Literature: Vol 2*. (Rev. ed). John Keats, 1795–1821 (III. 449–III. 459). Glenview, IL: Scott, Foresman.

Angier, N. (1997, April 3). Survey of scientists find a stability of faith in God. *New York Times*, p. A10.

Antoni, M.H., Baggett, L., Ironson, G., et al. (1991). Cognitive-behavioral stress management intervention buffered distress responses and immunologic changes following notification of HIV-1 seropositivity. *Journal of Consulting and Clinical Psychology, 59*, 906–915.

Antonovsky, A. (1979). *Health, Stress, and Coping: New Perspectives on Mental and Physical Well-Being*. San Francisco: Jossey-Bass.

Antonovsky, A. (1987). *Unraveling the Mystery of Health: How People Manage Stress and Stay Well*. San Francisco: Jossey-Bass.

Antonovsky, A. (1992). Can attitudes contribute to health? *Advances, 8*(4), 33–49.

Artress, L. (1995). *Walking a Sacred Path: Rediscovery of the Labyrinth as a Spiritual Tool.* New York: Riverhead Books.

Augros, R.M., & Stanciu, G.N. (1984). *The New Story of Science: Mind and the Universe.* Lake Bluff, IL: Regnery Gateway.

Ayto, J. (1990). *Arcade Dictionary of Word Origins.* New York: Little, Brown.

Azar, B. (1996, November). Some forms of memory improve as people age. *American Psychology Association Monitor,* p. 27.

Baker, C. (Ed.). (1981). *Ernest Hemingway, Selected Letters, 1917–1961.* New York: Charles Scribner's Sons.

Barsky, A.J., Cleary, P.D., & Klerman, G.L. (1992). Determinants of perceived health status of medical outpatients. *Social Science & Medicine, 34*(10), 1147–1154.

Bauby, J-D. (1997). *The Diving Bell and the Butterfly.* (J. Leggatt, Trans.). New York: Knopf.

Beecher, H.K. (1955). The powerful placebo. *Journal of the American Medical Association, 159*(17), 1602–1606.

Bellah, R., Madsen, R., Sullivan, W., Swidler, A., & Tipton, S. (1985). *Habits of the Heart: Individualism and Commitment in American Life.* Berkeley: University of California Press.

Bellow, S. (1997, May 27). Interviewed by M. Gussow. For Saul Bellow at 81, seeing with fresh eyes. *New York Times,* B1, B7.

Benner, P., & Wrubel, J. (1989). *The Primacy of Caring.* Menlo Park, CA: Addison-Wesley.

Benor, D.J. (1990, September). Survey of spiritual healing research. *Complementary Medical Research, 4*(1), 9–33.

Benor, D.J. (1993). *Healing Research.* Munich: Helix Verlag GmbH.

Benson, H. (1995). Commentary: Placebo effect and remembered wellness. *Mind/Body Medicine, 1*(1), 44–45.

Benson, H. (1996). *Timeless Healing: The Power and Biology of Belief.* New York: Scribner.

Benson, H., & Epstein, M.D. (1975). The placebo effect: A neglected asset in the care of patients. *Journal of the American Medical Association, 232*(12), 1225–1227.

Benson H., & Friedman, R. (1996). Harnessing the power of the placebo effect and renaming it remembered wellness. *Annual Review of Medicine, 47,* 193–99.

Berendt, J.E. (1987). *Nada Brahma: The World of Sound.* Rochester, VT: Destiny Books.

Blau, J.N. (1985). Clinician and placebo. *Lancet, 8424,* 344.

Block, K.I. (1997). The role of the self in healthy cancer survivorship: A view from the front lines of treating cancer. *Advances, 13*(1), 16–26.

Blum, A. (1997, April 15). Seeing patients—the sketchiest details. Presentation at the Health Care and Arts Lecture Series, University of Texas–Houston Health Science Center.

Bolen, J.S. (1996). *Close to the Bone: Life-Threatening Illness and the Search for Meaning.* New York: Scribner.

Booth, L. (1990). *Say Yes to Life.* Deerfield Beach, FL: Health Communications.

Bracke, P.E., & Thoresen, C.E. (1996). Reducing Type A behavior patterns: A structured group approach. In R. Allan & S. Scheidt (Eds.), *Heart & Mind: The Practice of Cardiac Psychology* (pp. 255–290). Washington, DC: American Psychological Association.

Breznitz, S. (1983). Denial versus hope: Concluding remarks. In Breznitz, S., (Ed.), *The Denial of Stress.* New York: International Universities Press.

Brody, H. (1977). *Placebos and the Philosophy of Medicine.* Chicago: University of Chicago Press.

Brody, H. (1987). *Stories of Sickness.* New Haven, CT: Yale University Press.

Brody, J.E. (1996a, February 28). Good habits outweigh genes as key to a healthy old age. *New York Times,* p. B9.

Brody, J.E. (1996b, February 28). Survivor enjoys her life at 83. *New York Times,* p. B9.

Brooks, R.T. (1989). *Ask the Bible.* New York: Gramercy Publishing.

Broyard, A. (1992). *Intoxicated with my Illness: And Other Writings on Life and Death.* New York: Clarkson Potter.

Buber, M. (1969). *The Legends of the Baal-shem*. New York: Schocken Books.

Buber, M. (1987). *I and Thou*. Second Edition. (R.G. Smith, Trans.). New York: Collier Books.

Buchholz, W.M., & Buchholz, S.W. (1997, January). *Conquering Fear*. Monograph. Mountain View, CA.

Buckman, R. (1992). Humankind is preset to value life. In Wholey, D. *When the Worst That Can Happen Already Has*. New York: Hyperion.

Buechner, F. (1992). *Listening to Your Life: Daily Meditations with Frederic Buechner*. San Francisco: HarperSanFrancisco.

Buechner, F. (1996). *The Longing for Home*. San Francisco: HarperSanFrancisco.

Bulman, J.R., & Wortman, C.B. (1977). Attributions of blame and coping in the "real world": Severe accident victims react to their lot. *Journal of Personality and Social Psychology, 35,* 351–363.

Byock, I. (1997). *Dying Well: The Prospect for Growth at the End of Life*. New York: Riverhead Books.

Cannon, W.B. (1942). "Voodoo" death. *American Anthropologist, 44*(2), 169–181.

Carter, B.J. (1991). Long-term survivors of breast cancer: A qualitative descriptive study. *Cancer Nursing, 16*(5), 354–361.

Carver, R. (1989). *A New Path to the Waterfall: Poems*. New York: Atlantic Monthly Press.

Cassell, E.J. (1982). The nature of suffering and the goals of medicine. *New England Journal of Medicine, 306,* 639–645.

Caudill, M.A. (1995). *Managing Pain Before It Manages You*. New York: Guilford Press.

Cheyne, J. (1983). *Guide to the Keats-Shelley Memorial House*. Piazzadi Spagna, Rome: Keats-Shelley Memorial Association.

Chopra, D. (1991). *Perfect Health*. New York: Harmony Books.

Claypool, J. (1992, January 27–28). Expectations, mercy and hope. Presentations at The Church of St. John the Divine, Houston.

Clearman, R. (1996, April 11). Dancing to survive. Health Care and the Arts Lecture Series. University of Texas-Houston Health Science Center.

Cohen, S. (Speaker). (1993). *On the Edge of Being: When Doctors Confront Cancer.* (Videocassette). Cerenex Pharmaceuticals.

Cohen, S.R., & Mount, B.M. (1992). Quality of life in terminal illness: Defining and measuring subjective well-being in the dying. *Journal of Palliative Care, 8*(3). 40–45.

Cousins, N. (1989). *Head First: The Biology of Hope.* New York: Dutton.

Cousins, N. (1990, March 29). New dimensions in healing. *President's Lecture Series.* University of Houston, Houston, TX.

Cowart, D. (1996, September 13). Presentation at Baylor College of Medicine. Compassion and the Art of Medicine Lecture Series, Houston.

Csikszentimihaly, M. (1990). *Flow: The Psychology of Optimal Experience.* New York: Harper.

Cushman, R.C., Jones, S. R., with Knopf, J. (1993). *Boulder County Nature Almanac.* Boulder, CO: Pruett.

Damasio, A.R. (1994). *Descartes' Error: Emotion, Reason, and the Human Brain.* New York: Putnam.

Damasio, H., Grabowski, T., Frank, R., Galabarda, A.M. & Damasio, A.R. (1994). The return of Phineas Gage: Clues about the brain from the skull of a famous patient. *Science, 264,* 1102–1105.

Dannen, K., & Dannen, D. (1981). *Rocky Mountain Wildflowers.* Estes Park, CO: Tundra Publications.

Delbruck, M. (1971). Aristotle-totle-totle. In J. Monod & E. Boreles, (Eds.). *Of Microbes and Life.* New York: Columbia University Press.

Dienstfrey, H. (1992). What makes the heart healthy? A talk with Dean Ornish. *Advances, The Journal of Mind-Body Health, 8*(2), 25–45.

Dillard, A. (1988). *Pilgrim at Tinker Creek.* New York: HarperPerennial.

Dimsdale, J. E. (1974). The coping behavior of Nazi concentration camp survivors. *American Journal of Psychiatry, 131*(7), 793–794.

Dimsdale, J.E., & Baum, A., (Eds.). (1995). *Quality of Life in Behavioral Medicine Research.* Hillsdale, NJ: Lawrence Erlbaum.

Ditto, P.H., Druley, J.A., Moore, K.A., Danks, J.H., & Smucker, W.D. (1996). Fates worse than death: The role of valued life activities in health-state evaluations. *Health Psychology, 15*(5), 332–343.

Dobyzhansky, T. (1967). *The Biology of Ultimate Concern.* New York: American Library.

Donnelley, D. (1982). *Putting Forgiveness into Practice.* Allen, TX: Argus Communications.

Dossey, L. (1984). *Beyond Illness: Discovering the Experience of Health.* Boston: New Science Library.

Dossey, L. (1991). *Meaning & Medicine.* New York: Bantam Books.

Dossey, L. (1993). *Healing Words: The Power of Prayer and the Practice of Medicine.* San Francisco: HarperCollins.

Dossey, L. (1994). *Power of Prayer, How to Pray and What to Pray For.* Tape 11280A-1. Niles, IL: Nightingale-Conant Corp.

Dossey, L. (1995). What does illness mean? *Alternative Therapies in Health and Medicine, 1*(3), 6–10.

Dossey, L. (1996, November/December). Healing happens. *Medicine & Prayer,* p. 3.

Druss, R.G., & Douglas, C.J. (1988). Adaptive responses to illness and disability. *General Hospital Psychiatry, 10,* 163–168.

Eliot, R.S., & Breo, D.L. (1984). *Is It Worth Dying For?* New York: Bantam Books.

Eliot, T.S. (1963). The dry salvages, V. *T.S. Eliot Collected Poems: 1909–1962* (pp. 191–199). New York: Harcourt, Brace, & World.

Ellis, H. (1923). *The Dance of Life.* Boston: Houghton Mifflin.

Ellison, C., Smith, J. (1991). Toward an integrative measure of health and well-being. *Journal of Psychology and Theology, 19*(1), 35–48.

Ephron, L., as quoted in L. Dossey. (1991). *Meaning & Medicine* (p. 139). New York: Bantam Books.

Erikson, E.H. (1963). The Golden Rule in the cycle of life. In R.W. White (Ed.), *The Study of Lives.* New York: Atherton Press.

Fant, III, J.L., & Ashley, R., (Ed.). (1964). *Faulkner at West Point.* New York: Random House.

Feifel, H. (1969). Attitudes toward death: A psychological perspective. *Journal of Consulting and Clinical Psychology, 33,* 292–295.

Feifel, H. (1990, April). Psychology and death. *American Psychologist, 45*(4), 537–543.

Ferguson, E. (1996, April). Memory of wellness: Our secret resource. Interview with Herbert Benson. *Brain/Mind Bulletin,* p. 5.

Feuerstein, M., Labbé, E.E., & Kuczmierczyk, A.R. (1986). *Health Psychology: A Psychobiological Perspective.* New York: Plenum Press.

Field, T. (1993, September). Volunteer grandparents may benefit more from massaging others than from receiving massage themselves. *Alternative Medicine,* p. 3.

Field, T., Schanberg, S.M., Scafidi, F., Bauer, C.R. Vega-Lahr, N., Garcia, R., Nystrom, J., & Kuhn, C.M. (1986). Tactile/kinesthetic stimulation effects on preterm neonates. *Pediatrics, 77*(5), 654–658.

Fine, S.B. (1991). Resilience & human adaptability: Who rises above adversity? *American Journal of Occupational Therapy, 456,* 493–503.

I Corinthians 12:26. *Holy Bible: The New King James Version (1984).* Nashville: Thomas Nelson Publishers.

I Corinthians 15:48–49. *Holy Bible: New International Version* (1987). Carmel, NY: Guideposts.

Fordyce, W.E. (1988). Pain and suffering: A reappraisal. *American Psychologist, 43*(4), 276–283.

Fordyce, W. E., Brockway, J.A., Bergman, J.A., & Spengler, D. (1986). Acute back pain: A control-group comparison of behavioral-traditional management methods. *Journal of Behavioral Medicine, 9*(12), 127–140.

Frank, A.W. (1991). *At the Will of the Body: Reflections on Illness.* Boston: Houghton Mifflin.

Frank, A.W. (1995). *The Wounded Storyteller: Body, Illness, and Ethics.* Chicago: University of Chicago Press.

Frankl, V. (1963). *Man's Search for Meaning.* (I. Lasch, Trans.). New York: Pocket Books.

Frankl, V. (1996, Winter). Address to the evolution of psychotherapy conference, Hamburg, Germany, July 1994. As presented in the *Milton H. Erickson Foundation Newsletter,* pp. 1, 18–20.

Freeman, L. (1989). *Light Within*. New York: Crossroad.

Freeman, L. (1994). *Everyday Spirituality*. Rydalmere, Australia: Hunt & Thorpe.

Freeman, L. (1996). *A Short Span of Days*. Ottawa, Canada: Novalis.

Freud, S. (1955). *Civilization and Its Discontents*. (J. Riviere, Trans.) London: Hogarth Press.

Friedman, M., Fleishman, N. & Price, V.A. (1996). Diagnosis of Type A behavior pattern. In R. Allan, S. Scheidt (Eds.), *Heart and Mind: The Practice of Cardiac Psychology* (pp. 179–195). Washington, DC: American Psychological Association.

Friedman, M., Powell, L.H., Thoresen, C.E., Ulmer, D., Price, V., Gill, J.J., Thompson, L., Rabin, D.D., Brown, B., Breall, W.S., et al. (1987). Effect of discontinuance of type A behavioral counseling on type A behavior and cardiac recurrence rate of post myocardial infarction patients. *American Heart Journal, 114*(3), 483–90.

Friedmann, E., Katcher, A.H., Lynch, J.J., & Thomas, S.A. (1980, July–August). Animal companions and one-year survival of patients after discharge from a coronary care unit. *Public Health Reports, 95*(4), 307–312.

Friedmann, E., Katcher, A.H., Thomas, S.A., Lynch, J.J., & Messent, P.R. (1983). Social interaction and blood pressure: Influence of animal companions. *Journal of Nervous & Mental Disease, 171*(8), 461–465.

Friend, D., & the Editors of *Life*. (1991). *The Meaning of Life*. Boston: Little Brown.

Fries, J.F., & Crapo, L.M. (1981). *Vitality and Aging*. New York: W.H. Freeman.

Fryback, P.B. (1993). Health for people with a terminal diagnosis. *Nursing Science Quarterly, 6*(3), 147–159.

Gallagher, T. (1989). Introduction. In R. Carver, *A New Path to the Waterfall: Poems* (pp. xvii–xxxi). New York: Atlantic Monthly Press.

Garraty, J.A., & Gay, P., (Eds.). (1987). *The Columbia History of the World*. New York: Harper & Row.

Gazzaniga, M.S. (1988). *Mind Matters: How Mind and Brain Interact to Create our Conscious Lives*. Boston: Houghton Mifflin.

Goethals, G.A., & Strauss, J.A., (Eds.). (1991). *The Self: Interdisciplinary Approaches*. New York: Springer-Verlag.

Goleman, D. (1996, February 26). Studies suggest older minds are stronger than expected. *New York Times,* p. A1.

Gomes, P. (1996). *The Good Book.* New York: William Morrow.

Goodare, H. (1997). A comment from an English cancer survivor. *Advances, 13*(1), 33–36.

Goodwin, J.S., Hunt, W.C., Key, C.R., & Samet, J.M. (1987). The effect of marital status on stage, treatment, and survival of cancer patients. *Journal of American Medical Association, 253*(21), 3125–3130.

Gordon, J. (1993, June 23). Practice of mind/body health care. Presentation at annual conference of Institute of Noetic Sciences, Arlington, Virginia.

Gould, K.L., Ornish, D., Scherwitz, L., Brown, S., Edens, R.P., Hess, M.J., Mullani, N., Bolomey, L., Dobbs, F., Armstrong, W.T., et al. (1995). Changes in myocardial perfusion abnormalities by positron emission tomography after long-term, intense risk factor modification. *JAMA 274*(11), 894–901.

Gussow, M. (1997, May 26). Interview. For Saul Bellow at 81, seeing with fresh eyes. *New York Times,* B1, B7.

Hagelin, J.S. (1983). *An Introduction to Unified Field Theories.* Fairfield, IA: Mill Press.

Hahn, R.A. (1984). Rethinking "disease" and "illness." In E.V. Daniel, & J. Pugh, (Eds.), *Contributions to Asian Studies: Special Volume on Southasian Systems of Healing, 18,* 1–23.

Hahn, R.A. (1995). *Sickness and Healing: An Anthropological Perspective.* New Haven, CT: Yale University Press.

Hammond, M. (1996, April 23). Music and spiritual anguish. Presentation at the Health Care & the Arts Lecture Series. University of Texas–Houston Health Science Center, School of Public Health.

Hanson, R.W. (1990). *Coping with Chronic Pain.* New York: Guilford Press.

Hardy, A. (1975). *The Biology of God: A Scientist's Study of Man the Religious Animal.* New York: Taplinger.

Harman, W. (1997, Spring). Biology revisioned. *Noetic Sciences Review,* pp. 12–17, 39–42.

Hay, D. (1982). *Exploring Inner Space: Scientists and Religious Experience*. London: Penguin Books.

Healthy People 2000: National Health Promotion and Disease Prevention Objectives. (1991). U.S. Department of Health and Human Services. Washington DC: U.S. Government Printing Office.

Healthy People 2000: Midcourse Review and 1995 Revisions. (1995). U.S. Department of Health and Human Services. Washington, DC: U.S. Government Printing Office.

Hebrews 11:1. *Holy Bible: The New King James Version* (1984). Nashville: Thomas Nelson Publishers.

Heisenberg, W. (1974). *Across the Frontier*. (P. Heath, Trans.). New York: Harper & Row.

Henneman, D. (1996, July/August). Praying with strangers. *Medicine & Prayer*, p. 2.

Henrich, E., & Kriegel, L. (1961). *Experiments in Survival*. New York: Association for the Aid of Crippled Children.

Hillman, J. (1993, November 18). Keynote address. American Art Therapy Association, Atlanta, GA.

Hirshberg, C., & Barasch, M.I. (1995). *Remarkable Recovery*. New York: Riverhead Books.

Hope, D. (1987). The healing paradox of forgiveness. *Psychotherapy, 24*, 240–244.

Horrigan, B. (1995a). Interview with Dean Ornish: Healing the heart, reversing the disease. *Alternative Therapies in Health and Medicine, 1*(5), 84–92.

Horrigan, B. (1995b). Interview with Candace Pert, Ph.D.: Neuropeptides, AIDS, and the science of mind-body healing. *Alternative Therapies in Health and Medicine, 1*(3), 70–76.

House, J.S., Landis, K.R., & Umberson, D. (1988). Social relationships and health. *Science, 241*, 540–545.

Idler, E.L. (1993). Perceptions of pain and perceptions of health. *Motivations and Emotion, 17*(3), 205–223.

Idler, E.L. (1995). Religion, health, and nonphysical senses of self. *Social Forces, 74*(2), 683–704.

Idler, E.L., & Angel, R.J. (1990). Self-rated health and mortality in the NHANES-I epidemiologic follow-up study. *American Journal of Public Health, 80*(4), 446–452.

Idler, E.L., & Kasl, S.V. (1991). Health perceptions and survival: Do global evaluations of health status really predict mortality? *Journal of Gerontology, 46*(2), S55–S65.

Idler, E.L., & Kasl, S.V. (1992). Religion, disability, depression, and the timing of death. *American Journal of Sociology, 97*(4), 1052–79.

Isaiah 40:11. *Holy Bible: The New King James Version* (1984). Nashville: Thomas Nelson Publishers.

Jaffe, A., (Ed.). (1979). *C. G. Jung: Word and Image.* Princeton, NJ: Princeton University Press.

James, J. & James, M. (1991). *A Passion for Life: Psychology and the Human Spirit.* New York: Dutton.

Janoff-Bulman, R., & Timko, C. (1987). Coping with traumatic life events. In Snyder, C.R. and Ford, C.E. (Eds.), *Coping With Negative Life Events: Clinical and Social Psychological Perspectives* (pp.135–159). New York: Plenum.

Jenkins, J.S. (1989, January 24). Coping with tragedy. Presentation at the Church of St. John the Divine, Houston.

Johns Hopkins Medical Letter: Health After 50. (1997, July). Heart disease: The mind-body connection.

Johnson, M.M. (1997, April 26). She's surviving—and thriving. *Houston Chronicle,* pp. 1E, 3E.

Jung, C.G. (1931/1962). Commentary. In R. Wilhelm, (C.F. Baynes, Trans.). *The Secret of the Golden Flower* (pp. 81–137). San Diego: Harcourt Brace.

Jung, C.G. (1965). In A. Jaffe, (Ed.), *Memories, Dreams, Reflections* (R. Winston & C. Winston, Trans.). New York: Vintage Books.

Justice, B. (1988). *Who Gets Sick: How Beliefs, Moods, and Thoughts Affect Health.* Los Angeles: Jeremy P. Tarcher (New York: Putnam).

Justice, B. (1994). Critical life events and the onset of illness. *Comprehensive Therapy, 20*(4), 232–238.

Justice, B. (1996, October 30). Meaning and measure of health in medically ill persons who perceive themselves as well. Institute Lecture Series. University of Texas–Houston Medical School.

Justice, B. (1997, May 13–14). Cognitive restructuring in heart disease and cancer. Seventh Annual Peete Memorial Lecture; Cognitive restructuring in making hearts healthy. Peete Memorial Grand Rounds. Trinity Lutheran Hospital, Kansas City, MO.

Kabat-Zinn, J. (1990). *Full Catastrophe Living*. New York: Dell.

Kalfon, E. (1991, Winter). Pets make a difference in long-term care. *Perspectives, 15*(4), 3–6.

Kaplan, G., Barell, V., & Lusky, A. (1988). Subjective state of health and survival in elderly adults. *Journal of Gerontology: Social Sciences, 43,* S114–S120.

Kaplan, G.A., & Camacho, T. (1983). Perceived health and mortality: A nine-year follow-up of the human population laboratory cohort. *American Journal of Epidemiology, 117*(3), 292–304

Kaplan, R.M. (1995). Quality of life, resource allocation, and the U.S. health-care crisis. In J.E. Dimsdale & A. Baum (Eds.), *Quality of Life in Behavioral Medicine Research* (pp. 3–30). Hillsdale, NJ: Lawrence Erlbaum Associates.

Kark, J.D., Shemi, G., Friedlander, Y., Martin, O., Manor, O., & Blondheim, S.H. (1996). Does religious observance promote health? Mortality in secular vs. religious kibbutzim in Israel. *American Journal of Public Health, 86*(3), 341–346.

Kasl, S.V., & Cobb, S. (1966). Health behavior, illness behavior, and sick-role behavior: II. *Archives of Environmental Health, 12,* 531–541.

Kass, L. (1988a, October 6). Interview transcript. Part I by B. Moyers on *The World of Ideas,* p. 2.

Kass, L. (1988b, October 7). Interview transcript. Part II by B. Moyers on *The World of Ideas,* pp. 4–5.

Kawaga-Singer, M. (1993). Redefining health: Living with cancer. *Social Science & Medicine, 37*(3), 295–404.

Keats, J. (1818). Endymion. In G.K. Anderson & R. Warnock (Eds.), *The World in Literature: Vol 2.* (Rev. ed.). (p. III: 452). Glenview, IL: Scott, Foresman.

Keats, J. (1820). To Autumn. *Op. cit.* (p. III: 459).

Keller, E.F. (1983). *A Feeling for the Organism: The Life and Work of Barbara McClintock*. New York: W.H. Freeman.

Klein, D.C. (1988). The power of appreciation. *American Journal of Community Psychology, 16*(3), 305–324.

Kliever, L.D. (1989). Preface. In L. D. Kliever, (Ed.), *Dax's Case: Essays in Medical Ethics and Human Meaning* (pp. xi–xvii). Dallas: Southern Methodist University Press.

Kobasa, S.C. (1979). Stressful life events, personality, and health: An inquiry into hardiness. *Journal of Personality and Social Psychology, 37*(1), 1–11.

Koenig, H. (1995, April 21). Spirituality and Aging. Paper presented at the conference on Spiritual Dimensions in Clinical Research, National Institute for Healthcare Research, Leesburg, VA.

Koenig, H.G., Cohen, H.J., George, L.K., Hays, JC., Larson, D.B., & Blazer, D.G. (1997). Attendance at religious services, Interleukin-6, and other biological parameters of immune function in older adults. *International Journal of Psychiatry in Medicine, 27* (3), 233–250.

Kolata, G. (1996, February 27). New era of robust elderly belies the fears of scientists. *New York Times*, p. A1.

Kosambi, D.D. (1967). Living prehistory in India. *Scientific American, 216*(2), pp. 105–114.

Krauss, P., & Goldfischer, M. (1990). *Why Me?* New York: Bantam Books.

Kübler-Ross, E. (1970). *On Death and Dying.* New York: Macmillan.

Kutner, N.G. (1994). Assessing end-stage renal disease patients' functioning and well-being: Measurement approaches and implications for clinical practice. *American Journal of Kidney Diseases, 24*(2), 321–333

Lafuma, L., (Ed.). (1963). *Oeuvres Completes.* (D.B. Morris, Trans.). Paris: Seuil. (Includes Pascal's prayer for good use of sickness).

Langer, E.J. (1989). *Mindfulness.* Reading, MA: Addison-Wesley.

Langer, E.J., & Rodin, J. (1976). The effects of choice and enhanced personal responsibility for the age: A field experiment in an institutional setting. *Journal of Personality and Social Psychology, 34,* 191–198.

Larson, D. (1995, April 21). Spiritual dimensions in clinical research. Paper presented at conference of National Institute for Healthcare Research, Leesburg, VA.

Larson, J.L., & Witham, L. (1997). Scientists are still keeping the faith. *Nature, 386,* 435–436.

Lawlis, G.F. (1996a). *Transpersonal Medicine: A New Approach to Healing Body-Mind-Spirit.* Boston: Shambhala.

Lawlis, G.F. (1996b, August 1). Transpersonal imagery, suffering, and pain. Presentation at Transpersonal Psychology seminar, Monterey, California.

Lawlor, B. (1996, October 31). Physical challenge opened doors to recovery. Breast cancer: A survivor's story. *Mountain-ear,* p. 20.

L'Engle, M. (1980). *Walking on Water: Reflections on Faith and Art.* Wheaton, IL: Harold Shaw.

Lerner, Max. (1990). *Wrestling With the Angel: A Memoir of My Triumph Over Illness.* New York: Norton.

Lerner, Michael. (1994). *Choices in Healing.* Cambridge, MA: MIT Press.

LeShan, L. (1994). *Cancer as a Turning Point.* Revised Edition. New York: Plume.

Levine, S. (1990, Spring). Interview. *Inquiring Mind, 6*(2), 1–6.

Lock, M. (1980). The organization and practice of East Asian medicine in Japan: Continuity and change. *Social Science & Medicine, 14B,* 245–253.

Locke, T. (1997, March 18). Interview with Jirka Rysavy. The man who made Corporate Express. *Boulder Daily Camera,* pp. 1D, 14D–16D.

Lovallo, W.R. (1997). *Stress & Health: Biological and Psychological Interactions.* Thousand Oaks, CA: Sage.

Lusseyran, J. (1959). *Le Monde Commence Aujourd'Hui.* Paris: La Table Ronde.

Lynch, J.J. (1977). *The Broken Heart: The Medical Consequences of Loneliness.* New York: Basic Books.

Maer, S., Leventhal, H., & Johnson, M., (Eds.). (1992). Self-assessed health and mortality: A review of studies. *International Review of Health Psychology.* New York: John Wiley.

Main, J. (1981). *Word Into Silence.* New York: Paulist Press.

Mairs, N. (1986). *Plaintext: Deciphering a Woman's Life.* New York: Perennial Library.

Mallon, T. (1997, June 15). In the blink of an eye. *New York Times Book Review*, pp. 10,12.

Mark 9:24. *Holy Bible: Revised Standard Version* (1984). Nashville: Thomas Nelson Publishers.

Marwick, C.(1995). Should physicians write "prayer" or "more frequent participation in religious observances" when prescribing for their patients? *JAMA, 273*(20), 1561–1562.

Mathew, R. (1995, April 22–23). Spirituality and substance abuse. Presentations at National Institute for Healthcare Research conference on Spiritual Dimensions in Clinical Research, Leesburg, VA.

Matlin, M. (1991). A reflection: In D. Friend & the Editors of *Life*. *The Meaning of Life* (p. 95). Boston: Little, Brown.

Matter, J.A. (1974). *Love, Altruism, and World Crisis: The Challenge of Pitirim Sorokin.* Chicago: Nelson-Hall.

Mattlin, B. (1996, May 5). Dr. Kevorkian, what about aiding "disposable" disabled? *Houston Chronicle,* p. 4C.

May, G.G. (1988). *Addiction and Grace.* San Francisco: Harper & Row.

Mayer, S. (1989). Wholly life: A new perspective on death. *Holistic Nursing Practice, 3*(4), 72–80.

Mayne, S. (1997, April 12). Westminster Abbey: Reflections. Presentation at Christ Church Cathedral, Houston.

McCraty, R., Atkinson, M., Tiller, W.A., Rein, G., & Watkins, A.D. (1995). The effects of emotions on short-term power spectrum analyses of heart rate variability. *American Journal of Cardiology, 76*(14), 1089–1093.

McCraty, R., Atkinson, M., & Tiller, W. (1995). New electrophysiological correlates associated with intentional heart focus. *Subtle Energies, 4*(3), 251–268.

McEntyre, M.C. (1995). A place to put the pain: Three cancer stories. *Literature and Medicine, 14*(1), 87–104.

McHugh, P.R. (1997, Winter). The Kevorkian epidemic. *American Scholar, 66*(1), 15–27.

Medalie, J.H., & Goldbourt, U. (1976). Angina pectoris among 10,000 men, II: Psychosocial and other risk factors. *American Journal of Medicine, 60,* 910–921.

Mellen, B. (1996, December 16). Doctors having more faith in prayer to help heal sick. *Houston Chronicle,* p. 9A.

Melzack, R. (1992, April). Phantom limbs. *Scientific American,* pp. 120–126.

Merchant, J.H. (1991). January. In *Daily Guideposts.* Carmel, NY: Guideposts, p. 7.

Messereni, P. (1984, June). Panel on pets as social support. Presentation at the Pacific Division of the American Association for the Advancement of Science, San Francisco.

Messervy, J.M. (1995). *The Inward Garden.* Photographs by Sam Abell. Boston: Little, Brown.

Methodist Times: Medical Staff. (1995, June 23). View through camera's lens offers new eye on disease, p. 2/2.

Meyer, C. (1991). *Surviving Death.* Mystic, CT: Twenty-third Publications.

Meyer, D.J. (1993). Lessons learned: Cognitive coping strategies of overlooked family members. In A.P. Turnbull, et al., (Eds.), *Cognitive Coping, Families, and Disability* (pp. 81–93). Baltimore: Paul H. Brookes Publishing.

Miller, A. (1991, February, 3). Interview. CBS *Sunday Morning.*

Miller, L. (1984). *On Top of the World.* Seattle: The Mountaineers.

Miller, T. (1995). *How to Want What You Have.* New York: Holt.

Mishlove, J. (1989). Spirituality and psychology: An interview with Frances Vaughan. *Noetic Sciences Review,* Spring, pp. 4–9.

Mishra, R.S. (1962). *The Textbook of Yoga Psychology.* New York: Julian Press.

Mitchell, E., & Williams, D. (1996, Summer). Book Review. The way of the explorer: An Apollo astronaut's journey through the material and mystical worlds. *Noetic Sciences Review,* p. 40.

Monsaingeon, B. (1988). *Mademoiselle: Conversations with Nadia Boulanger.* (R. Marsach, Trans.). Boston: Northeastern University Press.

Montagu, A. (1942). *How to Find Happiness and Keep It.* Garden City, NY: Doubleday Doran.

Moore, J.A. (1989). *You Can Get Bitter or Better*. Nashville: Abington.

Moore, N.G. (1996). Spirituality in medicine. *Alternative Therapies in Health and Medicine, 2*(6), 24–26, 103–105.

Mora, P. (1963). Urge and molecular biology. *Nature, 199*(4890), 212–219.

Morris, D.B. (1991). *The Culture of Pain*. Berkeley: University of California Press.

Morris, D.B. (1995, November/December). Why my pain is not your pain. *Arthritis Today*, pp. 18–24.

Mossey, J.M., & Shapiro, E. (1982). Self-rated health: A predictor of mortality among the elderly. *American Journal of Public Health, 72*(8), 800–808.

Mount, B.M. (1993, October 28). Compassion and the Art of Medicine Lecture Series. Baylor College of Medicine, Houston.

Mount, B.M. (1996a). Foreword. In L. Freeman. *A Short Span of Days* (pp. 7–8). Ottawa, Canada: Novalis.

Mount, B.M. (1996b, November 13). Transformations: Meditation as a way of living and dying. Presentation at symposium, Christ Church Cathedral, Houston.

Moyers, B. (1982). *Six Great Ideas: Beauty*. Interview with Mortimer Adler. Transcript of WNET/13 broadcast, New York.

Murphy, R.F. (1987). *The Body Silent*. New York: Henry Holt.

Murphy, R.F., Sheer, J., Murphy, Y., & Mack, R. (1988). Physical disability and social liminality: A study in the rituals of adversity. *Social Science & Medicine, 26*(2), 235–242.

Myers, D.G. (1992). *The Pursuit of Happiness: Discovering the Pathway to Fulfillment, Well-Being, and Enduring Personal Joy*. New York: Avon Books.

Nelson, K. (1996, July 10). Personal communication.

Newman, M.A. (1986). *Health As Expanding Consciousness*. St. Louis: Mosby.

Nucho, A.O. (1988). *Stress Management: The Quest for Zest*. Springfield, IL: Charles C Thomas.

Nuland, S. (1994). *How We Die: Reflections on Life's Final Chapter*. New York: Knopf.

Okun, M.A., Stock, W.A., Haring, M.J., & Witter, R.A. (1984). Health and subjective well-being: A meta-analysis. *International Journal of Aging and Human Development 19*(2), 111–131.

Olman, M. (1995, July 14). Luncheon presentation at The Hospice at the Texas Medical Center, Houston.

Ornish. D. (1990). *Reversing Heart Disease*. New York: Ballantine Books.

Ornish, D. (1993). Can lifestyle changes reverse coronary heart disease? *World Review of Nutrition & Dietetics, 72*, 38–48.

Ornish, D. (1995, November). Interviewed by B. Horrigan. Healing the heart, reversing the disease. *Alternative Therapies in Health and Medicine, 1*(5), 84–92.

Ornish, D. (1996). Foreword. In R. N. Remen. *Kitchen Table Wisdom*. New York: Putnam.

Ornish, D. (1997, January 31). Presentation on whether changes in lifestyle can reverse cancer as well as heart disease. University of California, San Francisco.

Palmer, D. (1988). *Looking at Philosophy*. Mountain View, CA: Mayfield Publishing.

Parks, L.B. (1997, April 26). Paradise lost. *Houston Chronicle*, pp. 1D, 10D.

Parsons, T. (1958). Definitions of health and illness in the light of American values and social structure. In E.G. Jaco, (Ed.). *Patients, Physicians and Illness*. Glencoe, IL: Free Press.

Pascal, B. (1966). The wager. *Pensées*. (A.J. Krailsheimer, Trans.). Middlesex, England: Penguin Books.

Patel, C., & Marmot, M.G. (1987). Stress management, blood pressure, and quality of life. *Journal of Hypertension, 5*, S21–28.

Patrick, D.L., & Erickson, P. (1993). *Health Status and Health Policy: Quality of Life in Health Care Evaluation and Resource Allocation*. New York: Oxford University Press.

Peete, D.C. (1990, May 15). A commentary on "hope," Trinity Lutheran Hospital, Kansas City, Missouri.

Pennebaker, J.W. (1990). *Opening up: The healing power of confiding in others*. New York: William Morrow.

Pennebaker, J.W. (1995). An overview. In J.W. Pennebaker (Ed.), *Emotion, Disclosure and Health*. Washington, DC: American Psychological Association.

Persinger, M.A. (1987). *Neuropsychological Bases of God Beliefs*. New York: Praeger.

Pert, C. (1995). Interviewed by B. Horrigan. Neuropeptides, AIDS, and the science of mind-body healing. *Alternative Therapies in Health and Medicine, 1*(3), 70–76.

Petit, C. (1996, January 21). A soldier in the war on AIDS. *San Francisco Chronicle,* pp. 1,3.

Phillips, D.P., & King, E.W. (1988). Death takes a holiday: Mortality surrounding major social occasions. *The Lancet, 2,* 728–732.

Phillips, D.P., Ruth, T.E., & Wagner, L.M. (1993). Psychology and survival. *The Lancet, 342,* 1142–1145.

Phillips, D.P., & Smith, D.G. (1990). Postponement of death until symbolically meaningful occasions. *JAMA, 263*(14), 1947–1951.

Polanyi, M. (1962). *Personal Knowledge.* Chicago: University of Chicago Press.

Post-White, J. (1993). The effects of imagery on emotions, immune function, and cancer outcome. *Mainlines, 14*(1), 18–20.

Price, R. (1994). *A Whole New Life: An Illness & A Healing.* New York: Plume.

Raver, A. (1994, December 29). When hope falters, balm for the soul. *New York Times,* p. C1.

Reifman, A. (1995). Social relationships, recovery from illness, and survival: A literature review. *Annals of Behavioral Medicine, 17*(2), 124–131.

Rein, G., Atkinson, M., & McCarty, R. (1995). The physiological and psychological effects of compassion and anger. *Journal of Advancement in Medicine, 8*(2), 87–105.

Remen, R.N. (1988, Autumn). Spirit: Resource for healing. *Noetic Sciences Review,* pp. 5–9.

Remen, R.N. (1996). *Kitchen Table Wisdom.* New York: Riverhead Books.

Remen, R.N. (1997, February 1). How stories heal. Presentation at Commonweal Conference on New Directions in Health and Healing, Bolinas, CA.

Reynolds, P., & Kaplan, G.A. (1990). Social connections and risk of cancer: Prospective evidence from the Alameda County study. *Behavioral Medicine, 16*(3), 101–110.

Richardson, M.A., Post-White, J., Grimm, E.A., Moye, L.A., Singletary, S.E., & Justice, B. (1997). Coping, life attitudes, and immune responses to imagery and group support after breast cancer treatment. *Alternative Therapies in Health and Medicine, 3*(5), 62–70.

Riley, J.F., Ahern, D.K., & Follick, M.J. (1988). Chronic pain and functional impairment: Assessing beliefs about their relationship. *Archives of Physical and Medical Rehabilitation, 69,* 579–582.

Rimer, S. (1995, September 11). Lovers of beauty sing a collective ode to Keats. *New York Times,* p. A8.

Rinpoche, S. (1992). *The Tibetan Book of Living and Dying.* New York: HarperSan-Francisco.

Roberts, Alan H. (1995). The powerful placebo revisited: Magnitude of nonspecific effects. *Mind/Body Medicine 1*(1), 35–43.

Robertson, G. (1996, April 26). Personal communication.

Robertson, J. (1990). *The Magnificent Mountain Women: Adventures in the Colorado Rockies.* Lincoln: University of Nebraska Press.

Rosenberg, E.S., Billingsley, J.M., Caliendo, A.M., et al. (1997). Vigorous HIV-1-specific CD4+ T cell responses associated with control of viremia. *Science, 278,* 1447–1450.

Roush, W. (1997). Herbert Benson: Mind-body maverick pushes the envelope. *Science, 276,* 357–359.

Rowland, J. (1997, February 1). Developments in psychooncology research. Commonweal Conference on New Directions in Health and Healing, Bolinas, CA.

Rysavy, J. (1997, March 18). Interviewed by T. Locke. The man who made Corporate Express. *Boulder Daily Camera,* pp. 1D, 14D–16D.

Sachs, O. (1987). *The Man Who Mistook His Wife for a Hat.* New York: Harper & Row.

Sachs, O. (1990). *Awakenings: Revised Edition.* New York: HarperCollins.

Sachs, O. (1991). Neurology and the soul. In P. Corsi (1991). *The Enchanted Loom: Chapters in the History of Neuroscience* (pp. 366–370). New York: Oxford University Press.

St. George, A., & McNamara, P.H. (1984). Religion, race and psychological well-being. *Journal for the Scientific Study of Religion, 23*(4), 351–363.

Scheier, M.F., & Carver, C.S. (1985). Optimism, coping, and health: Assessment and implication of generalized outcome expectancies. *Health Psychology, 4*, 219–247.

Scherwitz, L., McKelvain, R., Laman, C., Patterson, J., Dutton, L., Yusim, S., Lester, J., Kraft, I., Rochelle, D., & Leachman, R. (1983). Type A behavior, self-involvement, and coronary atherosclerosis. *Psychosomatic Medicine, 45*, 47–56.

Schlitz, M.J., & Lewis, N. (1996, Summer). The healing powers of prayer. *Noetic Sciences Review*, pp. 30–31.

Schmidt, R.M. (1993). Health Watch: Health promotion and disease prevention in primary care. *Methods of Information Medicine, 32,* 245–248.

Seale, A. (1997, May/June). Sipping tea with Ilya Prigogine, professor of physics, Nobel laureate. *Texas Alcade,* pp. 24–29.

II Corinthians 5:7. *Holy Bible: New Revised Standard Version* (1989). New York: Oxford University Press.

Seligman, M.E.P. (1988, October). Boomer blues. *Psychology Today.* pp. 50–55.

Seligman, M.E.P. (1989). Research in clinical psychology: Why is there so much depression today? In I.S. Cohen, (Ed.), *The 1988 G. Stanley Hall Lecture Series* (pp. 79–96). Washington, DC: American Psychological Association.

Seligman, M.E.P. (1991). *Learned Optimism.* New York: Knopf.

Shakespeare, W. (1955a). The third part of King Henry the Sixth. II.ii.68. *The Histories and Poems of Shakespeare.* Vol. III. (1595). Chicago: Spencer Press.

Shakespeare, W. (1955b). King Lear. V.ii. *The Tragedies of Shakespeare* (1608). Chicago: Spencer Press.

Shakespeare, W. (1955c). Troilus and Cressida. III.iii.146–148. *The Tragedies of Shakespeare* (1609). Chicago: Spencer Press.

Sharkey, F. (1982). *A Parting Gift.* New York: St. Martin's.

Sheed, W. (1989, December). Making the spiritual connection. *Lears,* p. 73.

Sheldrake, R. (1985). *A New Science of Life: The Hypotheses of Formative Causation.* London: Blond, & Briggs.

Sheldrake, R. (1994, Summer). Opening up to the "numinous." *Noetic Science Review,* pp. 6–7.

Shepherd, G.M. (1994). *Neurobiology*. New York: Oxford University Press.

Shuman, R. (1996). *The Psychology of Chronic Illness*. New York: Basic Books.

Siegel, B.S. (1986). *Love, Medicine, & Miracles*. New York: Harper & Row.

Sigerist, H.E. (1941). *Medicine and Human Welfare*. New Haven: Yale University.

Singer, K. (1996, May–June). A conversation on faith. *Medicine & Prayer*, p. 2.

Smith, Huston. (1986). *The Religions of Man*. New York: Harper & Row.

Snyder, C.R., & Ford, C.E., (Eds.) (1987). Coping with traumatic life events. In *Coping With Negative Life Events: Clinical and Social Psychological Perspectives* (pp. 135–159). New York: Plenum.

Sorokin, P.A. (1964). *The Basic Trends of Our Times*. New Haven: College and University Press.

Spiegel, D. (1993). *Living Beyond Limits*. New York: Fawcett Columbine.

Spiegel, D., Bloom, J. R., Kraemer, H.C., & Gottheil, E. (1989). Effect of psycho-social treatment on survival of patients with metastatic breast cancer. *The Lancet, 2*, 888–91.

Stapp, H.P. (1993). *Mind, Matter & Quantum Mechanics*. Berlin: Springer-Verlag.

Sternberg, E.M. (1997). Emotions and disease: From balance of humors to balance of molecules. *Nature Medicine, 3*(3), 264–267.

Stevens, W.K. (1993, November 30). Want a room with a view? Idea may be in the genes. *Science Times*, pp. B5, B9.

Stronck, D. (1997, April 26). Interviewed by L.B. Parks. Paradise lost. *Houston Chronicle*, pp. 1D, 10D.

Styron, William. (1990). *Darkness Visible: A Memoir of Madness*. New York: Random House.

Suchman, A.L., & Matthews, D.A. (1988). What makes the patient–doctor relationship therapeutic? Exploring the connexional dimension of medical care. *Annals of Internal Medicine, 108*, 125–130.

Taylor, S.E. (1989). *Positive Illusions: Creative Self-deception and the Healthy Mind*. New York: Basic Books.

Taylor, S.E. (1995). *Health Psychology*. Third Edition. New York: McGraw-Hill.

Taylor, S.E., & Aspinwall, L.G. (1990). Psychological aspects of chronic illness. In G. R. VandenBos, & P.T. Costa, Jr. (Eds.), *Psychological Aspects of Serious Illness*. Washington, DC: American Psychological Association.

Taylor, S.E., Kemeny, M.E., Reed, G.M., & Aspinwall, L.A. (1991). In G.A. Goethals, & J.A. Strauss (Eds.), *The Self: Interdisciplinary Approaches* (pp. 239–254). New York: Springer-Verlag.

Taylor, S.E., Lichtman, R.R., & Wood, J.V. (1984). Attributions, beliefs about control, and adjustment to breast cancer. *Journal of Personality and Social Psychology, 46,* 489–502.

Tempellar, R., De Haes, J.C.J.M., De Ruiter, J.H., Bakker, D., Van Den Heuvel, W.J.A., & Van Nieuwenhuijzen, M.G. (1989). The social experiences of cancer patients under treatment: A comparative study. *Social Science & Medicine, 295*(5), 635–642.

Tetrault, D. (1997, June 29). Sermon on the healing of Jairus's daughter, Grace Episcopal Church, Yorktown, VA.

Thomas, L. (1992). *The Fragile Species*. New York: Charles Scribner.

Thoreau, H.D. (1960). *Thoreau on Man & Nature*. Mount Verson, NY: Peter Pauper Press.

Thoresen, C.E. (1989, August 13). Counseling and Type A: Issues of Assessment, Treatment, and Conceptualization. Paper presented at the 97th Annual American Psychological Association meeting, New Orleans.

Thorne, B. (1993, June 25). Discussant at presentation by Caryle Hirshberg on cancer remission project. Institute of Noetic Sciences Conference, Crystal City, VA.

Tillich, P. (1952). *The Courage to Be*. New Haven, CT: Yale University Press.

Topf, L.N., with Bennett, H.Z. (1995). *You Are Not Your Illness*. New York: Simon & Schuster.

Topping, A.D. (1997, June 22). A miracle called Charlie. *Houston Chronicle*, pp. 1F, 9F.

Treaster, J.B. (1997, March 26). Finding ability, not just disability. *New York Times,* pp. C1, C4.

Trillin, A.S. (1981). Of dragons and garden peas: A cancer patient talks to doctors. *New England Journal of Medicine, 304*(12), 699–701.

Turnbull, A. P., Patterson, J.M., Behr, S. K., Murphy, D.L., Marquis, J.G., & Blue-Banning, M.J., (Eds.). (1993). *Cognitive Coping, Families, and Disability.* Baltimore: Paul H. Brookes Publishing.

Tye, L. (1997, November 22). New treatment in early stages of AIDS gives hope of extending lives. *Houston Chronicle,* p. 18 A.

Vaillant, G.E. (1977). *Adaptation to Life.* Boston: Little, Brown and Company.

Vaillant, G.E., & Vaillant, C.O. (1990). Natural history of male psychological health, XII: A 45-year study of predictors of successful aging at age 65. *American Journal of Psychiatry, 147*(1), 31–37.

VandenBos, G.R., & Costa, P.T. Jr. (Eds.). *Psychological Aspects of Serious Illness.* Washington, DC: American Psychological Association.

Veatch, V. (1997, January 31). The Ting-sha cancer help program. Commonweal Conference on New Directions in Health and Healing, Bolinas, CA.

Verbrugge, L.M., & Balaban, D.J. (1989). Patterns of change in disability and well-being. *Medical Care, 27*(3Suppl), S128–S147.

Wakefield, D. (1996). *Creating From the Spirit.* New York: Ballentine.

Walsh, A., & Walsh, P.A. (1989). Love, self-esteem, and multiple sclerosis. *Social Science & Medicine, 29*(7), 793–798.

Watson, J. (1968). *The Double Helix.* New York: Mentor.

Watts, A. (1996). *Buddhism: The Religion of No Religion.* Boston: Charles E. Tuttle.

Wedemeyer, D. (1996, August 18). His life is his mind. *New York Times Magazine,* pp. 22–25.

Wheeler, J.A. (1977). Genesis and observership. In R.E. Butts & J. Hintikka (Eds.). *Problems in the Special Sciences* (pp. 5–6). Dordrecht, Holland: Reidel.

Wholey, D. (1992). *When the Worst That Can Happen Already Has.* New York: Hyperion.

Williams, R. (1989). *Trusting Heart.* New York: Times Books.

Williams, R.B., Barefoot, J.D., Califf, R.M., Haney, T.L., Saunders, W.B., Pryor, D.B., Hlatky, M.A., Siegler, I.C., & Mark, D.B. (1992). Prognostic importance of social and economic resources among medically treated patients with angiographically documented coronary artery disease. *JAMA, 267*(4), 520–524.

Wolf, S. (1959). The pharmacology of placebos. *Pharmacological Reviews, 11*, 689–704.

Wordsworth, W. Lines composed a few miles above Tintern Abbey, on revisiting the banks of the Wye during a tour (1798). In *The Poetical Works of Wordsworth* (pp. 114–115). London: Frederick Warne and Co. (publication date not given).

Wordsworth, W. Intimations of immortality from recollections of early childhood (1807). In *The Poetical Works of Wordsworth* (pp. 313–317). London: Frederick Warne and Co. (publication date not given).

World Health Organization. (1947). Annex I: Constitution of the world health organization. In *Chronicle of the World Health Organization*. New York: World Health Organization Interim Commission.

Zajonc, R.B. (1985). Emotion and facial efference: A theory reclaimed. *Science, 228*(4695), 15–21.

Zwinger, A., & Willard, B. (1972). *Land Above the Trees: A Guide to American Alpine Tundra.* Tucson: University of Arizona Press.

Acknowledgments

I am particularly grateful to Gail Bray, Jennifer Le,

Carol Busby, Kimberly Nelson, and my wife, Rita, for helping

make this book a reality. It also would have not been possible

without the willingness and cooperation of the women

I interviewed from the breast cancer project. I give them

heartfelt thanks for the time they spent with me.

INDEX

A

abdominal cancer, 114–15
accomplishment, 106, 170, 201, 218
Adams, John, 169
adaptation, 62–63, 64
adventures, 208, 214–215, 230
adversity, 53, 163, 201, 219
aesthetics, 117
affective indifference, 39–40
to affiliate, 99, 109
Affleck, Glenn, 50, 54
aging
　ingredients of successful, 204–5
　outlook vs. genes and, 208–10
　resilience and, 210–12
　See also longevity
AIDS, 1, 45, 47, 65, 213
Albert Einstein Medical School, 65
alchemy, 62, 64, 109, 119, 201, 249
alcohol, 45, 180, 223, 244
Alcoholics Anonymous, 180
Alfieri, Vittorio, 139
ALS (Lou Gehrig's disease), 63, 151–52
altruism. *See* service
altruistic atheists, 269n.15
Alzheimer's disease, 77
American Academy of Family Physicians, 189
American Academy of Hospice and Palliative Medicine, 230
American Association for the Advancement of Science, 89–90
American Journal of Public Health, 188
Amsterdam Avenue (NYC), 85, 110, 246, 247
A, Mrs., 215–16

anencephaly, 102–3
anger, 40, 93, 101, 122, 123–25, 132, 145, 192–93, 222
　See also emotions
animals, 206–8, 269–70n.21
Anna, 65
Annals of Internal Medicine, 57
anniversary, 6, 168
antidepressants, 180
Antonovsky, Aaron, 61, 101
anxiety, 33, 171, 222, 227
Apollo 14 mission, 178
appreciation
　of beauty, 122–23
　cancer patients and, 111–12
　of the distinct in life, 108–9
　for escape from death, 116
　of the good in life, 107–8
　learning, 97–98
　for love, 114
　See also gratitude
appreciation research, 103–4
Arab Proverb, 225
Aristotle, 55, 78, 80, 117–18, 176
Army War College, 159
ars moriendi, 237
　See also dying well
art, 120, 136–37, 170, 171, 262n.16
arthritis, 10
ashes, 180, 193, 208, 245
asthma, 137, 220
astonishment, 99–100
atheists, 182, 269n.15
atherosclerosis, 73
athletes, 71, 153, 166, 235

A NOTE ON THE TYPE

———————————✺———————————

This book is set in Adobe Bembo,
which is based on an original cut by Francesco Griffo.
Bembo was first used in 1495 by printer-publisher
Aldus Manutius for *De Aetna* by Cardinal Bembo,
whom the modern version is named after.

ABOUT THE AUTHOR

Blair Justice, Ph.D., is a Professor of Psychology at the University of Texas-Houston Health Science Center, School of Public Health, where he also serves as Associate Dean for Academic Affairs. He is the author of numerous papers in the scientific literature and four other books (two with his wife, Dr. Rita Justice). His 1988 book, *Who Gets Sick: How Beliefs, Moods, and Thoughts Affect Health,* has been published in four languages. At the School of Public Health, in collaboration with M.D. Anderson Cancer Center, Dr. Justice directed a pioneering pilot study comparing the effects of imagery, support, and standard care on immune function and psychosocial measures in women who had completed treatment for breast cancer. He is a co-investigator of the University of Texas Center for Alternative Medicine Research in Cancer and a Visiting Scholar at the University of Colorado in Boulder. Before becoming a psychologist, Dr. Justice was a science writer on metropolitan newspapers.

He and his wife are avid hikers and mountain climbers as well as longtime joggers. They both do volunteer service at The Hospice at the Texas Medical Center.